Complementary & Alternative Medicine (CAM) Supplement Use in People with Diabetes:
A CLINICIAN'S GUIDE

Chemical constituents, mechanism of action, adverse effects, and drug interactions for 36 commonly used supplements.

Laura Shane-McWhorter, PharmD, BCPS, FASCP, BC-ADM, CDE

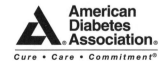

American Diabetes Association

Cure • Care • Commitment®

Managing Editor, Book Publishing, Abe Ogden; *Acquisitions Editor, Professional Books,* Victor Van Beuren; *Editor,* Aime Ballard-Wood; *Production Manager,* Melissa Sprott; *Composition,* Aptara, Inc.; *Cover Design,* pixiedesign, llc; *Printer,* Transcontinental Printing.

Printed in Canada
1 3 5 7 9 10 8 6 4 2

The suggestions and information contained in this publication are generally consistent with the *Clinical Practice Recommendations* and other policies of the American Diabetes Association, but they do not represent the policy or position of the Association or any of its boards or committees. Reasonable steps have been taken to ensure the accuracy of the information presented. However, the American Diabetes Association cannot ensure the safety or efficacy of any product or service described in this publication. Individuals are advised to consult a physician or other appropriate health care professional before undertaking any diet or exercise program or taking any medication referred to in this publication. Professionals must use and apply their own professional judgment, experience, and training and should not rely solely on the information contained in this publication before prescribing any diet, exercise, or medication. The American Diabetes Association—its officers, directors, employees, volunteers, and members—assumes no responsibility or liability for personal or other injury, loss, or damage that may result from the suggestions or information in this publication.

⊗ The paper in this publication meets the requirements of the ANSI Standard Z39.48-1992 (permanence of paper).

ADA titles may be purchased for business or promotional use or for special sales. To purchase more than 50 copies of this book at a discount, or for custom editions of this book with your logo, contact Lee Romano Sequeira, Special Sales & Promotions, at the address below, or at LRomano@diabetes.org or 703-299-2046.

For all other inquiries, please call 1-800-DIABETES.

American Diabetes Association
1701 North Beauregard Street
Alexandria, Virginia 22311

Library of Congress Cataloging-in-Publication Data

Shane-McWhorter, Laura.
   Complementary and alternative medicine (CAM) supplement use in people with diabetes / Laura Shane-McWhorter.
       p. ; cm.
   Includes bibliographical references and index.
   ISBN 978-1-58040-296-5 (alk. paper)
   1. Diabetes–Alternative treatment.   2. Dietary supplements.   I. American Diabetes Association.   II. Title.
   [DNLM: 1. Diabetes Mellitus–therapy.   2. Complementary Therapies–methods.
3. Dietary Supplements.   4. Plants, Medicinal. WK 815 S528c 2007]
   RC661.A47S53 2007
   616.4′6206–dc22

                                                                          2007014526

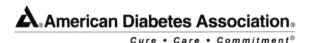

Contents

Acknowledgments

I would like to thank my family, friends, and support personnel, who have provided much encouragement, support, and counsel during my work on this book. Specifically, I would like to thank my husband, Jerry, as well as my children, Chris, Sandy, Randy, and David, and my grandson, Cody. I would like to give a special thank you to my friend Dick for his invaluable technical support.

Finally, I would also like to thank Victor Van Beuren of the American Diabetes Association, who believed this was a worthwhile endeavor.

1.

Introduction

Medical journals, the lay press, and the Centers for Disease Control and Prevention have highlighted the ever-increasing number of diabetes cases, now exceeding 20 million in the U.S.[1] Although there are numerous conventional, or allopathic, therapies to treat diabetes, there is also a tremendous interest in emerging therapies, including nontraditional, or complementary and alternative, medicine. Complementary and alternative medicine therapeutic modalities have become increasingly popular, and it is estimated that consumers spent $17.7 billion dollars on oral supplements in 2001.[2]

Two distinct definitions of these unique therapies are important for clinicians to differentiate. One is the definition of complementary and alternative medicine (CAM) and the other is the definition of dietary supplements. The National Center for Complementary and Alternative Medicine (NCCAM) has provided a definition of complementary and alternative medicine. NCCAM states that CAM therapies cover a broad range of healing philosophies, approaches, and treatments. CAM is defined by NCCAM as treatments and health care practices not widely taught in medical schools, not generally used in hospitals, and not usually reimbursed by insurance companies.[3] In CAM therapy, the health care practitioner considers the whole person, including not only physical, mental, and emotional characteristics, but also spiritual aspects. Hence the term "holistic" is used to characterize treatment. Some of these therapies are used alone and referred to as "alternative." Other therapies are combined with other alternative or conventional therapies and referred to as complementary.[3] NCCAM has categorized CAM into four different domains: biologically based therapies, mind-body medicine, energy medicines, and manipulation and body-based practices.

Biologically based therapies include the use of herbs and dietary supplements. Oral CAM therapies may include botanical products or nonbotanical products such as vitamins and minerals, and are sometimes referred to as "dietary supplements." A definition of dietary supplements has been provided by the Dietary Supplement Health and Education Act of 1994.[4] A dietary supplement is "a product taken by mouth that contains a 'dietary ingredient' intended to supplement the diet and may include vitamins, minerals, herbs or other botanicals, amino acids, enzymes or glandulars, or some type of concentrate, metabolite, or extract."[5]

Thus, CAM therapies have included dietary supplements (herbals and vitamins) and other treatments such as acupuncture, relaxation techniques, massage, chiropractic, and spiritual healing.[6] In diabetes, certain types of CAM therapies that have been considered useful include not only herbal and homeopathic products but also certain diets, acupuncture, energy healing, biofeedback, hypnotherapy, reflexology, massage therapy, and yoga.[7]

This book will use the term "CAM supplements" to describe nontraditional oral agents that are of botanical or nonbotanical origin. Hundreds of different plant species have been recorded as being useful to treat diabetes.[7,8] Indeed, metformin is a biguanide that is widely prescribed in patients with type 2 diabetes, and this class of agents is related to *Galega officinalis* L., or goat's rue,[9] which was used for many centuries to treat diabetes. There are also numerous nonbotanical products that patients have used to treat diabetes.

Unfortunately many clinical studies that have assessed the use of CAM supplements are limited in number or are fraught with design problems. Yet clinicians involved in the care of patients with diabetes often encounter patients who are using these supplements. Instead of simply telling patients not to use these products, it is important to respect the patient's health beliefs and address his or her questions in an unbiased manner. It is imperative that clinicians learn about CAM supplements their patients may be taking concurrently with prescribed medications for diabetes, related comorbidities, or other disease states. Clinicians may then advise their patients and discuss CAM product use in an open manner. Clinicians who provide medical care for diabetes patients must learn about the potential use, adverse effects, and drug-drug or drug-disease interactions produced by these supplements. It is also important for clinicians to access accurate sources to provide information to their patients. The intent of this book is to provide information that may help clinicians learn about CAM supplements often used by patients with diabetes. It is also important for clinicians to maintain an open mind and be considerate of their patients' wishes.

REASONS FOR CONCERN REGARDING CAM SUPPLEMENT USE

A primary reason to address CAM use by diabetes patients is that they are 1.6 times more likely than people without diabetes to use these treatments and hence may be more vulnerable to problems resulting from CAM supplement use.[10] Two potential concerns immediately emerge: side effects and drug interactions. Other concerns include variability of products, lack of standardization, contamination, and misidentification. Confusion regarding product content and labeling is another issue. A recent concern is whether clinical investigations actually verify the content of CAM supplements being studied.[11] Of equal concern is that there may be additional costs associated with CAM supplement use and may be delays in initiation of proven treatments.

A clinician may not even be aware that a patient is using CAM supplements. Less than 40% of patients tell their health care provider they are using CAM treatments.[6,12] A patient may experience a side effect that the provider may attribute to another medication, when in fact it could be due to a CAM supplement. Many serious side effects have been experienced by patients taking complementary therapies.[13,14] In individuals with diabetes, some products have caused irreversible hypoglycemia (*Amanita phalloides*) and critical hepatic glycogen depletion (unripe Ackee fruit).[8] Unorthodox practices to treat diabetes, such as urine treatment, have also been reported.[15] Clinicians should note that certain ethnic groups may be more reticent about reporting CAM supplement use to their health care providers.[15]

Potential drug interactions are another concern.[16,17] Since people with diabetes often have to take other medications, concomitant use of CAM supplements may result in toxicity secondary to exaggerated or subtherapeutic effects from their medications. For instance, ginseng may be used to treat diabetes, but may interfere with the ability of warfarin to produce its anticoagulant effect.[18] Alternatively, a product may produce a drug-disease interaction. For instance, ginseng may increase blood pressure.[19]

Another potential problem is untoward reactions during surgery, secondary to CAM supplement use. Some products may cause excessive bleeding during surgery or interact with anesthetics, and patients may experience increases or decreases in blood pressure.[20,21] Because patients do not normally consider CAM supplements to be actual drugs, they may not tell providers they are taking them, and therefore providers may not ask the patients to stop use before surgery.[20,21]

Product variability is another reason for caution. CAM supplements are available in a variety of forms, including tablets, capsules, or liquid extracts (if water-based they are called decoctions or infusions; if hydroalcoholic they are called tinctures). Alcohol-free glycerin-extracted preparations are called glycerites. The quality of a botanical product may depend on what part of the plant was used, how it was grown and stored, how long it was stored, how it was processed, and how the extract was prepared.[14] A group of investigators assessed 59 products containing Echinacea, as a single ingredient, available in a retail setting.[22] The investigators' intent was to determine whether the Echinacea species used was consistent with the labeled content. The researchers found that 52% (31 of 59) of products accurately reported the content, while 10% (6 of 59) contained no measurable Echinacea. For 18 samples where actual content differed from labeled content, 39% (7) contained more species than were listed on the label and 56% (10) contained fewer species. This is a prime example of product content variability. Hence it becomes very confusing for clinicians to determine which brand is most or least acceptable and what dose should be used.

Some products are available in standardized forms or standardized extracts. Ideally, standardization should guarantee consistency in each product batch as well as stability of the active ingredients. However, the active constituents are unknown for many agents, making standardization a difficult process. Furthermore, a botanical standardized constituent may show consistency between products, but may not necessarily be the active ingredient.[23] For instance, St. John's wort has two main marker constituents, hypericin and hyperforin. Many researchers believe that hyperforin may be the more active species in providing therapeutic effects.[24] But should the results of well-designed studies where hypericin was the standardized extract in a clinical investigation be ignored? Pharmacological action of CAM supplements may be due to combined effects of several ingredients, and the individual ingredients may not produce the same effects as the whole plant.[25] Active botanical constituents may vary because of differences in geographic location or soil conditions, exposure to rain or sun, harvest time, and processing methods (drying and storage). Thus, pharmacological activity may be affected.[26]

Other factors include potential misidentification, mislabeling, addition of unnatural toxic substances, such as heavy metals or steroids, and contamination with microbes, pesticides, fumigants, or radioactive products.[26] One example of contamination was the inadvertent substitution of *Aristolochia serpentaria* for *Stephania tetranda* in a weight-loss product, which resulted in Chinese herb nephropathy.[27] Another example was a dietary supplement available in American stores and by mail order, that was found to contain an unlabeled ingredient, glyburide, a prescription sulfonylurea.[28] Lead contamination of CAM products used to treat diabetes has also been reported.[29,30]

There are wide variations in CAM supplement product labels, which may also be very confusing. This issue has been addressed in different investigations. In one study the investigators assayed six bottles each of two different supplement lots from nine different manufacturers containing Echinacea, kava, saw palmetto, ginseng, and St. John's wort.[31] Labels for the same product from different manufacturers were inconsistent in recommended daily amounts and botanical information regarding species, plant part used, and marker compounds. The greatest variability in that study was found in products containing Echinacea and ginseng. For example, the Echinacea contained the purpurea, pallida, or angustifolia species separately or in combination. The Echinacea products may have been derived from the aerial parts or the root. For ginseng, measured amounts ranged from 44% to 261% of what was stated on the bottle. The researchers noted that products from the same manufacturer but different lots of the same plant contained different plant parts. The least bottle for bottle variability was found for saw palmetto, kava, and St. John's wort.

Another study assessed the label information of 10 popular herbs from 20 retail settings to determine consistency of reported ingredients and recommended daily doses.[32] The investigators found that labels for 43% of 880 (379) products were consistent in reported benchmark ingredients (benchmarked according to ingredients in a reputable dietary supplement text) and recommended daily doses. Only 20% (179) were consistent in ingredients but not recommended doses, and 37% (329) lacked consistency in reporting ingredients or had vague label information that rendered it impossible to assess ingredient information. These reports verify that there is great inconsistency and variability in labeled information.

Furthermore, many investigators do not evaluate the product contents when conducting a clinical study. A group of researchers analyzed randomized controlled trials published between 2000 and 2004 of single-ingredient products including Echinacea, garlic, ginkgo, saw palmetto, or St. John's wort to determine whether the investigators evaluated and verified the product content.[11] The investigators found that 15% (12 of 81 studies) reported performing tests to calculate actual product contents and only 4% (3 studies) provided sufficient data to compare actual and expected content values of at least one chemical ingredient. The investigators found that in those three studies actual constituent content ranged from 80% to 113% of expected values.

Yet another thing to consider is the potential increased indirect costs of diabetes, because individuals with diabetes may substitute ineffective complementary therapies or delay treatment with proven therapeutic agents. These costs may include increased hospitalizations, acute complications such as ketoacidosis or acute hyperglycemia, or chronic complications such as retinopathy.[33] Other potential costs include decreased work productivity and diminished ability to function in a social or occupational setting if patients are substituting less effective treatments for more effective therapies. Conversely, a recent study examined whether CAM users with diabetes neglected preventive health care maintenance practices. The study found that CAM use was correlated with increased preventive health practices, including pneumococcal immunizations and visits to primary care providers.[34]

EPIDEMIOLOGY OF CAM SUPPLEMENT USE

A landmark study in 1990 indicated that 33.8% of Americans use alternative medicine, although this included a variety of modalities such as acupuncture and chiropractic in addition to oral supplements.[6] The study was repeated in 1997, and researchers found that alternative medicine use had increased to 42.1%.[12] A finding with important ramifications from the latter survey was that 15 million adults take alternative agents concurrently with prescription drugs. This survey also found that 12.1% of patients take herbal supplements and 5.5% take megavitamins. A 2002 report of medication use in the U.S. indicated that herbals or supplements were used by 14% of the population surveyed.[35]

Information regarding how many patients with diabetes use CAM supplements has been elucidated by several recent studies. A recent publication reported information regarding CAM supplement use in diabetes patients, using data from the 2002 National Health Interview Survey (NHIS).[34] The NHIS included questions regarding CAM use and included data from approximately 2,500 people with diabetes. The researchers determined that 48% of individuals with diabetes reported using some type of CAM therapy, which included many different modalities.

Some of these modalities included acupuncture, Ayurveda, biofeedback, chelation, massage, naturopathy, special diets, and herbal therapies. According to the researchers analyzing the NHIS data, 22% of people with diabetes used some type of herbal therapy.

A study using 1996 Medical Expenditure Panel Survey data reported that people with diabetes are 1.6 times more likely than people without diabetes to use CAM (8% vs. 5%, $P < 0.0001$).[10] Nutritional advice and lifestyle diets were the most commonly used therapies. These included Ayurvedic diets, naturopathic or homeopathic nutrition diets, as well as orthomolecular therapies including melatonin, vitamin megadoses, or magnesium administered by CAM practitioners. Other modalities included spiritual healing, herbal remedies, massage therapy, and meditation training.

Other surveys of diabetes clinic patients indicate that 17% to 57% use CAM.[36–38] In one study 17% used CAM therapies. Acupuncture, homeopathy, and herbal therapy were used most often.[36] Another study found that 31% used dietary supplements.[37] The most commonly used supplements were garlic, Echinacea, herbal mixtures, glucosamine, chromium, ginkgo biloba, fish oil, cayenne, and St. John's wort.[37] Data from a national survey of CAM use found that in individuals with diabetes 57% had used CAM treatments in the past year.[38] Prayer and spiritual practices, herbal remedies, commercial diets, and folk remedies were reported most often.[38] A smaller percentage, 35%, reported use of products specifically for diabetes. Interestingly, patients with diabetes have felt that complementary therapies were useful, but less than their prescription medications.[37]

CAM therapy use in specific ethnic groups with diabetes has also been reported. In Navajos with diabetes 39% used CAM therapies,[39] in Hispanics with diabetes in South Texas 49% used CAM,[40] and in a Vietnamese population with diabetes two-thirds used CAM.[41] In an evaluation of a small sample of Hispanic diabetes patients, researchers found that most participants were taking both traditional folk remedies and conventional medications.[42] Some of the commonly used products included aloe vera (sábila) and prickly pear cactus (nopal).[42] Another important finding in this study of Hispanics, with important implications for clinicians, was that many of the participants believed that diabetes may be caused by fright (*susto*) or anger (*coraje*) and that insulin may cause blindness and become an addiction. Other surveys of Hispanic patients have found that folk remedies such as herbal teas or other botanical products were used by 33%[43] to 64%.[15] Unlike studies that have stated that <40% of patients reported use of CAM supplements to their provider,[6] studies in Hispanics have found that as many as 69% did not report use of herbal remedies.[15] Hence, clinicians should be more proactive in asking their Hispanic patients about CAM supplement use.

CAM supplement use has also been reported across several age groups. One study reported that dietary supplements were used by children with chronic diseases including asthma, cancer, cystic fibrosis, diabetes, hepatic or renal disorders, and rheumatology and neurobehavioral disorders.[44] In the children with diabetes, 31% were using a nonprescribed supplement.[44] On the opposite end of the age spectrum, a small multiethnic sample of older individuals found that 15% used herbal remedies and 5% used teas to treat their diabetes.[45] In female seniors who were members of a health plan, 11% of women with diabetes used herbal products.[46]

REGULATION OF CAM SUPPLEMENTS

Dietary supplements do not need FDA approval before being marketed.[4] Prior to 1994, CAM supplements were classified as foods or drugs, depending on the intended use. In 1994, Congress passed the Dietary Supplement Health and Education Act (DSHEA), which created a separate category for botanicals and other products.[47] Now they are classified as dietary supplements.[47] This legislation allows dietary supplements to forego the same stringent approval process that is required for drugs, and therefore proof of safety and efficacy is not required for marketing.

The reclassification has resulted in a serious consequence. Sometimes contaminants or substitutes have been found in the products. For instance, as noted above, some diabetes products have been contaminated with lead,[29,30] and other products touted as being "herbal" have been found to contain prescription drugs such as chlorpropamide or glyburide.[28,48]

A possible solution would be the use of standardized products. Standardization guarantees that each dose provides a consistent level of the active ingredient. However, proponents of biological complementary therapies argue that standardized extracts may not always contain all of the therapeutic ingredients found in the natural product. A pertinent factor is whether the standardized preparation actually reflects the labeled information.[22]

DSHEA allows manufacturers of dietary supplements to make claims regarding the ability to maintain "structure and function" of the body, but does not allow claims regarding diagnosis, treatment, cure, or prevention of disease.[47] If a manufacturer claims the product affects body structure or function, the label must include the following statement: "This statement has not been evaluated by the Food and Drug Administration (FDA). This product is not intended to diagnose, treat, cure, or prevent any disease." The manufacturer must also notify the FDA within 30 days after a product is on the market if it bears such a label.

FDA has implemented regulations that ban implied as well as expressed disease claims.[47] For example, claims made by a manufacturer that a patient could misconstrue as indicating treatment or prevention of a disease are no longer allowed. In the new regulations, a product may make health maintenance claims but not disease claims ("maintains a healthy prostate" is allowed, but "treats benign prostatic hyperplasia" is not).

FDA has published a Dietary Supplement Strategy (Ten Year Plan).[49] The year 2010 is the target year when FDA will have a "science-based regulatory program that fully implements DSHEA, in an effort to provide consumers with a high level of confidence in the safety, composition, and labeling dietary supplement products." This program will assist clinicians in providing better information to people with diabetes who use CAM supplements.

TESTING CAM SUPPLEMENTS

An unfortunate situation is that most consumers believe that dietary supplements are evaluated for content and efficacy by an appropriate regulatory agency. The Harris Poll conducted 1,010 telephone interviews with a cross-section of adults in October 2002. The poll indicated that 68% of Americans believe the government requires herbal manufacturers to report potential dangers or adverse effects.[50] Additionally, 58% believed that government agencies, such as the FDA, must approve herbal products before sale to the public, and 55% believed that manufacturers cannot make claims for supplement safety or efficacy without scientific evidence. Additionally, 13% believed that because supplements are "natural" they are safe.[50] Actually, supplement manufacturers, not the FDA, are responsible for determination of safety and veracity of label claims. Most individuals do not realize that manufacturers do not have to tell the FDA or consumers what evidence they have about supplement safety or to back up their claims.[51]

Accuracy of labeling and ingredient purity may now be assessed by different dietary supplement testing programs. Unfortunately, efficacy is not evaluated. An example of an organization that has established certification programs for dietary supplements is the U.S. Pharmacopeia (USP). The USP program is called the Dietary Supplement Verification Program.[52] The "USP-verified mark" on the label indicates the product ingredients are accurate and that the product is pure, will dissolve properly, and has been manufactured using good manufacturing practices. Clinicians should note that the USP website also lists manufacturers that have undergone the evaluation process.[52]

NSF International (formerly known as National Sanitation Foundation) also verifies products for label and content accuracy, checks purity and contaminants, and audits the manufacturing process for good manufacturing practice compliance.[53] Consumer Lab also tests supplements.[54] It tests certain classes for purity and accuracy of labeled ingredient content. All of these companies require that manufacturers pay for testing.[55] The Consumers Union also tests certain products and reports findings in their publication, *Consumer Reports*.[56] The National Nutritional Foods Association (NNFA) has also launched a good manufacturing practice program. Recently, NNFA changed its name to the Natural Products Association, and more information may be obtained at their website.[57]

EVALUATING CLAIMS FROM MANUFACTURERS OF DIETARY SUPPLEMENTS

Manufacturers may use deceptive marketing tactics to promote their products. Clinicians may wish to access the FDA website that provides suggestions on "How to Spot Health Fraud."[58] One caveat provided by the website is to be wary of a single product claiming benefit for a variety of unrelated diseases (for instance, difficulties ranging from menstrual problems to asthma to rheumatic complaints). Other caveats are to be wary of evidence of benefit based on personal testimonials, claims of unusually rapid benefit, or use of meaningless phrases that may sound scientifically impressive to lay consumers who do not have the education or training to determine veracity.

The FDA Center for Food Safety and Applied Nutrition has established two websites for consumers to evaluate information about dietary supplements. "Tips for the Savvy Supplement User"[59] includes basic points to consider, such as talking with a health care provider before using a supplement, broaching the issue that some supplements may interact with prescription or over-the-counter medicines or have untoward effects during surgery. It also provides information on how to report adverse effects of dietary supplements. Furthermore, it provides tips on searching the Web for information on dietary supplements, such as how to find out who operates the site, the purpose of the site, the information sources and references, and whether the information is current. Another website, "Tips for Older Dietary Supplement Users,"[60] discusses potential risks, such as the danger of substitution of dietary supplements for conventional medications or the dangers associated with consuming greater than recommended amounts. It also advocates discussion of dietary supplement use with the patient's health care provider. It provides a checklist of important considerations such as issues with side effects, drug interactions, and possible discontinuation before scheduled surgery.

The following includes excerpts from *The Health Professional's Guide to Popular Dietary Supplements*[61] and provides other information that may help clinicians:

- Nationally known companies generally have more stringent quality assurance and incorporate good manufacturing practices. Some companies may even import products tested in Europe. A list of these is included in *The Complete German Commission E Monographs: Therapeutic Guide to Herbal Medicines.*[62]
- The following questions may elucidate useful information when contacting a manufacturer:[61]
  - Has the product been evaluated in clinical studies published in peer-reviewed journals? If so, is the company willing to share these studies?
  - Can the manufacturer explain the pharmacological mechanism? Is there research to support this mechanism?
  - Does the company complete an analysis of the active as well as inert ingredients?
  - Does the company complete an analysis of the final product to insure that package contents match the labeled information?
  - Does the product meet bioavailability standards for disintegration dissolution?
  - What are the storage or stability precautions?
  - What are listed contraindications for product use?

CAM SUPPLEMENTS USED FOR DIABETES AND ITS COMPLICATIONS

Although there are hundreds of different botanical and nonbotanical products to treat diabetes and its complications, this book will focus on some of the most well-known and commonly used products, roughly in order of popularity. A discussion of botanical or dietary sources, chemical constituents and mechanism of action, adverse effects and drug interactions, examples of the types of clinical studies that evaluate these substances, and an overall summary will be presented for each product.

Botanical biological complementary therapies used to lower blood glucose include cinnamon (*Cinnamomum cassia*), gymnema (*Gymnema sylvestre* R.Br.), fenugreek (*Trigonella foenum-graecum*), bitter melon (*Momordica charantia*), ginseng (*Panax ginseng* or *Panax quinquefolius* L.), nopal (*Opuntia streptacantha*), aloe (*Aloe vera* L.), banaba (*Lagerstroemia speciosa* L.), caiapo (*Ipomoea batatas*), ivy gourd (*Coccinia indica*), holy basil (*Ocimum sanctum*), Vijayasar (*Pterocarpus marsupium* Roxb. [Leguminoceae]), jambolan (*Eugenia jambolana*), blonde psyllium (*Plantago ovata*), glucomannan (*Amorphophallus konjac* K. Koch), guar gum (*Cyamopsis tetragonolobus* [L.] Taub), stevia (*Stevia rebaudiana* Bertoni), pine bark (*Pinus pinaster*), and tea (*Camellia sinensis*), which may include green, oolong, or black tea. Claims have been made for bilberry (*Vaccinium myrtillus*) and milk thistle (*Silybum marianum*), but there is less evidence for these and other products.

Nonbotanical biological complementary supplements that may lower blood glucose include chromium, vanadium, nicotinamide, magnesium, and coenzyme Q10.

Botanical and nonbotanical products thought to decrease the complications of diabetes include the vitamin-like substance alpha-lipoic acid, vitamin E, gamma-linolenic acid, ginkgo (*Ginkgo biloba* L.), fish oil, policosanol (*Saccharum officinarum* L.), garlic (*Allium sativum*), guggul (*Commiphora mukul*), and red yeast rice (*Monascus purpureus* Went). Another biological complementary product frequently used is St. John's wort (*Hypericum perforatum* L.), which is used to treat some types of depression rather than diabetes. However, depression frequently occurs in diabetes patients and many clinicians consider this a complication of diabetes.

2.

Botanical CAM Supplements to Treat Diabetes

C AM supplements of botanical origin have been used to treat diabetes for many centuries. Although some products were once common only in certain parts of the world, their use has now become more mainstream. Many of the products originated in Asia and India and with time have been adopted in Europe and other parts of the Western world. Interest in the use of these substances has increased, and many have been evaluated in studies. This chapter will provide an overview of many of the botanical products used to treat diabetes. Table 1 (on page 75) provides a brief summary of the information in this section.

CINNAMON (*Cinnamomum cassia*)

Cinnamon is one of many complementary and alternative medicine (CAM) supplements that have been used to treat diabetes. It is one of several dietary supplements that fall under the legislation of the Dietary Supplement Health and Education Act of 1994.[4] Although cinnamon bark and cinnamon flower are used medicinally, Chinese cinnamon, or *Cinnamomum aromaticum* (synonym *C. cassia*), is the form used for diabetes. This product is also known as cassia.[63] Cinnamon comes from an evergreen tree that grows over 20 feet (up to 7 meters) high and has a white aromatic bark and angular branches. It has leaves about 7 inches (18 cm) long and small yellow flowers that bloom in early summer. The tree grows in tropical climates, and the bark is removed in short lengths and dried.[63]

Cinnamon has been used for type 2 diabetes and for gastrointestinal complaints such as dyspepsia or flatulence. Cinnamon is a popular flavoring agent in different foods and beverages and is a common ingredient in chewing gum, toothpaste, mouthwash, and other products.[19]

Chemical Constituents and Mechanism of Action

The active ingredient is thought to be hydroxychalcone, a polyphenolic polymer that may enhance the effect of insulin. Specifically, it may work on insulin receptors to increase insulin sensitivity, promote cell and tissue glucose uptake, and promote glycogen synthesis.[64]

Adverse Effects and Drug Interactions

Adverse effects include irritation or contact dermatitis, if used topically.[62] Allergic reactions may also occur. There are no reported drug interactions. In theory, cinnamon may lower blood glucose if combined with secretagogues such as sulfonylureas or insulin.

Clinical Studies

A study in Pakistan in 60 individuals with type 2 diabetes who were taking sulfonylureas found that cinnamon improved glucose and lipids.[65] Patients were given 1, 3, or 6 g/day cinnamon or placebo for 40 days. Fasting blood glucose declined by 18–29% after 40 days in all three groups. At a dose of 1 g/day, glucose decreased from a baseline of 209 mg/dl (11.6 mmol/l) to 157 mg/dl (8.7 mmol/l); at 3 g/day, glucose decreased from 205 mg/dl (11.4 mmol/l) to 169 mg/dl (9.4 mmol/l); and at 6 g/day, glucose decreased from 234 mg/dl (13.0 mmol/l) to 166 mg/dl (9.2 mmol/l) ($P < 0.05$ for all three groups vs. baseline). Cinnamon was withheld for the next 20 days, and fasting glucose was still lower than at baseline, indicating that cinnamon had a sustained benefit. Improvements in lipids were also significant. Total cholesterol decreased by 12–26%, triglycerides decreased by 23–30%, and LDL cholesterol also declined by 7–27% ($P < 0.05$ for all three parameters). HDL cholesterol did not improve, and the authors did not report changes in A1C.

Another study was done in Germany in 79 individuals with type 2 diabetes being treated with oral agents or diet.[66] This 4-month randomized double-blind, placebo-controlled trial evaluated use of an aqueous cinnamon extract, essentially devoid of coumarins (<0.1%) and thought to be less allergenic than other forms. Patients were randomized to a placebo or a capsule containing 1 g cinnamon three times a day. In the cinnamon group, mean baseline fasting glucose decreased from 167 mg/dl (9.3 mmol/l) to 147 mg/dl (8.2 mmol/l) after 4 months ($P < 0.001$). The placebo group had a decrease from mean baseline of 156 mg/dl (8.7 mmol/l) to 150 mg/dl (8.3 mmol/l; results not significant). The mean percentage difference was 10.3% in the treatment group and 3.37% in the placebo group ($P = 0.046$). Mean baseline A1C did not decrease significantly. Mean A1C declined from a baseline of 6.86% to 6.83% in the cinnamon group and from 6.71% to 6.68% in the placebo group. There were no differences in lipids. Mean baseline LDL cholesterol was 134 mg/dl (3.5 mmol/l) and 135 mg/dl (3.5 mmol/l) at end point in the cinnamon group. The mean baseline and end point LDL cholesterol did not change in the placebo group and was 138 mg/dl (3.6 mmol/l).

Summary

Research is currently underway to evaluate the effects of cinnamon in type 2 diabetes. The active ingredient is thought to be hydroxychalcone, which may enhance insulin sensitivity. Cinnamon decreases fasting glucose,[65, 66] and in one study total cholesterol, triglycerides, and LDL were also decreased.[65] A more recent study showed that in subjects with lower fasting glucose there was a significant decline, but there were no changes in A1C or lipids.[66] Differences in the two studies that are available seem to indicate that cinnamon may be more effective in individuals who have higher glucose values. Side effects are benign, and there are no known interactions, although doses of secretagogues may have to be adjusted to prevent hypoglycemia. Doses used in one study of subjects with high baseline glucose included 1, 3, or 6 g/day in divided doses.[65] Another study used 1 g three times a day of an aqueous cinnamon extract.[66] The amount used in studies is equivalent to about a half teaspoonful of ground cinnamon per day, which may be used in cereals, in beverages, on breads, and in other foods.

GYMNEMA (*Gymnema sylvestre* R. Br.)

Gymnema is a unique botanical product that has been used for centuries in Ayurvedic medicine. It is also known as *gurmar*, the "sugar destroyer," because it dulls the ability to taste "sweetness."[67] In India, gymnema has been traditionally used to treat *madhu meha*, "honey urine," or diabetes.[68] This woody climbing plant grows in tropical forests in central and southern India. The leaves are the part used for medicinal purposes.[69] Gymnema has been used in both type 1 and type 2 diabetes.

Chemical Constituents and Mechanism of Action

The constituents include a variety of chemicals, including saponins, stigmasterol, quercitol, the gymnemosides, and the amino acid derivatives betaine, choline, and trimethylamine.[70] Although the exact mechanism of action is unknown, varying effects from animal and in vitro cell research have shed light on how it may work. Gymnema appears to increase enzyme activity responsible for glucose uptake and use.[71] Gymnema may also stimulate pancreatic β-cell function, increase numbers of pancreatic β-cells, and possibly increase insulin release by increasing cell permeability to insulin.[68,69,72] For Gymnema to produce its pharmacological effects, some residual pancreatic function may be required, since in pancreatectomized animals it does not produce a hypoglycemic effect.[73] Work is continuing to elucidate more specific information on its pharmacological activity.

Adverse Effects and Drug Interactions

No adverse effects have been reported for gymnema, although in theory it may cause hypoglycemia. Gymnema may enhance the blood glucose lowering effects of certain drugs used to treat diabetes. These drugs include insulin, sulfonylureas, or the nonsulfonylurea secretagogues.

Clinical Studies

Gymnema has been researched since the 1930s.[68] In a study of 27 patients with type 1 diabetes, gymnema was administered at a dose of 200 mg twice a day for 6–30 months.[69] The researchers tracked A1C, fasting blood glucose, and insulin dose. Average A1C declined from 12.8% at baseline to 9.5% after 6–8 months ($P < 0.001$), and after 16–18 months 22 individuals continuing to take gymnema had a mean A1C of 9% (P values not stated). At the end of 26–30 months, six patients remaining on gymnema had a further decline to 8.2% (P values not stated). Average fasting glucose declined from 232 mg/dl (12.9 mmol/l) at baseline to 177 mg/dl (9.8 mmol/l) after 6–8 months, 150 mg/dl (8.2 mmol/l) after 16–18 months, and 152 mg/dl (8.4 mmol/l) after 20–24 months (P values not stated). Average insulin dose decreased from 60 units/day to 45 units/day after 6–8 months and declined further to 30 units/day after 26–30 months (P values not stated). A control group of 37 patients who took only insulin was also followed for 10–12 months, and these individuals had no change in blood glucose or A1C.

In a different study, 22 patients with type 2 diabetes took gymnema at a dose of 400 mg daily for 18–20 months in addition to a sufonylurea.[74] A1C declined from an average baseline of 11.9% to 8.5% ($P < 0.001$), and average fasting glucose decreased from 174 mg/dl (9.7 mmol/l) at baseline to 124 mg/dl (6.9 mmol/l) after 18–20 months ($P < 0.001$). Notably, five individuals were able to discontinue sulfonylurea treatment. Lipids also significantly declined in this study. A control group of 25 patients on sulfonylureas plus placebo had no significant changes in A1C, fasting glucose, or lipids.

Summary

Gymnema has been studied for up to 2 years in both type 1 and type 2 diabetes. Target goals for A1C and fasting glucose have not been achieved in published studies. Gymnema has a variety of actions that may stimulate glucose uptake and utilization as well as stimulate β-cell function. If gymnema is used, a standardized extract should be chosen. This product has not been studied in pregnant or lactating women, children, or elderly and therefore should not be used in these populations. The main potential adverse effect is hypoglycemia; hence it is important that medical providers supervise their patients' use of this product and possibly consider decreasing the dose of concomitant secretagogues. A standardized gymnema extract is being studied in the U.S. A typical dose is 400 mg/day, standardized to contain 24% gymnemic acids.[19]

FENUGREEK (*Trigonella foenum-graecum* L.)

Fenugreek is a member of the Leguminosae, or Fabaceae, family and grows well in India, Egypt, and other parts of the Middle East.[75] The leaves are ingested as a vegetable in India.[76] The part used medicinally is the seed.

Not only has fenugreek been used to treat diabetes, but since it tastes and smells like maple syrup, it has also been used as a cooking spice and flavoring agent in foods and tobacco. It has been used to mask the taste of medicines.[75] Other uses include treatment of constipation and hyperlipidemia, and postpregnancy use to promote lactation.[75] There are no studies supporting its use in lactation.

Chemical Constituents and Mechanism of Action

Fenugreek contains many different chemical components, including saponins and several glycosides.[75] The seeds contain alkaloids, including trigonelline, gentianine, and carpaine compounds. Fiber,

4-hydroxyisoleucine, and fenugreekine, components that may have hypoglycemic activity, are also found in the seeds. The mechanism is thought to involve delay of gastric emptying, slowing carbohydrate absorption, and inhibition of glucose transport.[77] Fenugreek may also increase the number of insulin receptors in red blood cells and improve glucose utilization in peripheral tissues; thus demonstrating potential antidiabetic effects in both the pancreas and other sites.[78] A constituent of the seeds, 4-hydroxyisoleucine, may directly stimulate insulin secretion.[79]

Adverse Effects and Drug Interactions

The main side effects include diarrhea and gas, or flatulence, which subside after a few days of use. A caution for women of childbearing age is that fenugreek consumption may cause uterine contractions and thus cause problems with pregnancy.[75] Hypersensitivity reactions have occurred, including rhinorrhea, wheezing, and fainting after inhalation of the seed powder. Wheezing and facial angioedema were reported in a patient with chronic asthma after application of a topical fenugreek paste.[76]

A theoretical adverse effect is an allergic reaction in people with a peanut allergy, since peanuts are also members of the Leguminosae family.[76] However, this reaction has never been reported. All of these side effects may occur in the infants of nursing mothers who use fenugreek, since the fenugreek may be secreted in the milk.

Fenugreek contains some coumarin constituents, and thus may increase the effects of anticoagulant, or blood-thinning, drugs such as warfarin (Coumadin) or herbs with blood-thinning activity (such as ginkgo biloba, garlic, or ginger). A case report of an interaction between warfarin and a product containing the digestive agent boldo in combination with fenugreek resulted in an increase in international normalized ratio (INR).[80] Fenugreek may also enhance the activity of diabetes medications; thus, when used in combination with insulin or oral diabetes agents, the patient may experience hypoglycemia.

Clinical Studies

There are only a few published studies using fenugreek. Most of these are short-term, involve very few patients, and do not adequately report details. In one study, 10 patients on insulin (with type 1 diabetes) were included in a 10-day evaluation.[81] The patients were assigned to either placebo or twice-daily 50 g fenugreek defatted seed powder, used in unleavened bread. Fasting glucose decreased from an average of 272 mg/dl (15.1 mmol/l) at baseline to 196 mg/dl (10.9 mmol/l; $P < 0.01$). Total cholesterol decreased ($P < 0.001$), as did LDL and triglycerides ($P < 0.01$ for both).

A larger study involved a 6-month trial of fenugreek in 60 patients with inadequately controlled type 2 diabetes.[82] Fenugreek seed powder, 25 g daily, was given in two equal doses at lunch and dinner. The average fasting glucose decreased from 151 mg/dl (8.4 mmol/l) to 112 mg/dl (6.2 mmol/l) after 6 months. Glucose values 1 and 2 hours after meals also declined. Mean baseline 1-hour glucose measured by oral glucose tolerance test (OGTT) was 245 mg/dl (13.6 mmol/l) at the start of the study and decreased to 196 mg/dl (10.9 mmol/l) after 6 months ($P < 0.001$). Mean 2-hour glucose decreased from 257 mg/dl (14.3 mmol/l) to 171 mg/dl (9.5 mmol/l; $P < 0.001$). Average A1C decreased from 9.6% to 8.4% after 8 weeks ($P < 0.001$).

In a different study, 25 newly diagnosed type 2 diabetes patients were given a hydroalcoholic fenugreek extract or placebo plus usual care of diet and exercise for 2 months.[83] The group assigned to fenugreek was given 1 g/day of the seed extract. The fenugreek group did not differ from the placebo group in fasting or postprandial glucose, although they had improved area under the curve blood glucose and insulin levels ($P < 0.001$) and an improved lipid profile for triglycerides and HDL.

Summary

In the U.S., fenugreek has GRAS (generally recognized as safe) status[84] and has been used in both type 1 and type 2 diabetes. However, there are few studies confirming its efficacy. It may have beneficial effects in pancreatic and other tissues and may affect glucose and carbohydrate absorption, as well as affect insulin resistance. Side effects are mostly uncomfortable gastrointestinal effects that may resolve in a few days. Pregnant women should not take fenugreek, since they may experience uterine contractions.[75] Women who use fenugreek as a galactogogue should be aware that it may appear in breast milk, and their infant may experience the side effects of this botanical. Caution is warranted in those who have a peanut allergy or are allergic to chickpeas, soybeans, or green peas. Individuals who take antiplatelet agents, anti-inflammatory drugs, or herbs that have blood-thinning effects should not use fenugreek. Although the dose used is variable, a typical amount is 10–15 g/day, as a single dose or divided with meals, or 1 g of a hydroalcoholic extract.[19] If fenugreek is combined with insulin or other diabetes medications, the patient may experience hypoglycemia; thus doses of diabetes medications may have to be adjusted.

BITTER MELON (*Momordica charantia*)

Bitter melon is a plant product also known as bitter gourd, bitter cucumber, and karela. It is a member of the Cucurbitaceae family and is related to honeydew and Persian melon, cantaloupe, muskmelon, and casaba. Although used for diabetes, bitter melon is cultivated in various parts of the world, including India, Asia, Africa, and South America, for consumption as a vegetable. Bitter melon grows as a vine with green leaves and yellow flowers. The fruit is green with a bumpy exterior, resembling a cucumber, and the interior is yellow-orange. The fruit and seeds are thought to be useful for diabetes.[75, 85]

Bitter melon has also been used for psoriasis, gastrointestinal disorders, kidney stones, and fever, and as a topical agent for wounds and abscesses. Women have used bitter melon to help induce menstruation and as an abortifacient. Recently it has also been used to treat cancer and HIV.[75, 85, 86]

Chemical Constituents and Mechanism of Action

Bitter melon contains several chemical ingredients, including the glycosides momordin and charantin. Polypeptide P, charantin, and vicine are the specific components thought to produce hypoglycemic effects.[75, 85] Other possible mechanisms in diabetes include increased tissue glucose uptake, increased liver/muscle glycogen synthesis, inhibition of enzymes involved in glucose production (glucose-6-phosphatase, fructose-1, and 6-bisphosphatase), and enhanced glucose oxidation (by the glucose-6-phosphate dehydrogenase, or G6PDH, pathway).[75, 85]

Adverse Effects and Drug Interactions

The major side effect of bitter melon is gastrointestinal discomfort. However, some very serious, isolated events have occurred, including hypoglycemic coma from a tea containing bitter melon. Another syndrome called favism, or hemolytic anemia, has occurred; it is characterized by headache, fever, abdominal pain, and coma. Individuals of Mediterranean or Middle-Eastern ancestry, who may have a G6PDH deficiency, may be prone to the hemolytic anemia. The red arils around the seeds have been reported to cause vomiting, diarrhea, and death in one child. Certain ingredients, α-momorcharin and β-momorcharin, are known abortifacients.[75, 85, 86]

When bitter melon is combined with sulfonylureas such as chlorpropamide (Diabinese), hypoglycemia may occur, and this has been reported.[87]

Clinical Studies

Few studies have evaluated bitter melon in diabetes, and most do not have adequate study design. The largest study used an aqueous suspension of bitter melon vegetable pulp in 100 patients with type 2 diabetes. The authors did not state the amount of bitter melon used, but stated it was based on body weight. On the first day, mean fasting blood glucose was 152 mg/dl (8.4 mmol/l); and after a 75-g OGTT, mean 2-hour postprandial glucose was 257 mg/dl (14.3 mmol/l). On day 2, mean fasting glucose was 160 mg/dl (8.9 mmol/l); then bitter melon extract was given, and mean blood glucose 1 hour later was 131 mg/dl (7.3 mmol/l; $P < 0.001$ vs. fasting value). A 75-g OGTT was then given, and mean 2-hour blood glucose was 222 mg/dl (12.3 mmol/l) (lower than the previous day's 2-hour value of 257 mg/dl [14.3 mmol/l], but not significant).[88]

In another study, bitter melon was prepared as an injectable "plant insulin" and injected in five patients with type 1 diabetes and six patients with type 2 diabetes. The dose used was based on blood glucose levels (10 units for blood glucose <180 mg/dl [<10.0 mmol/l], 20 units for blood glucose 180–250 mg/dl [10.0–13.9 mmol/l], 30 units for blood glucose >250 mg/dl [>13.9 mmol/l]). A control group consisted of six patients with type 1 diabetes and two patients with type 2 diabetes who did not receive any bitter melon. Fasting glucose was measured; then bitter melon was administered, and glucose was measured at 4, 6, 8, and 12 hours after injection. In patients with type 1 diabetes, mean fasting glucose decreased from 304 mg/dl (16.9 mmol/l) to 169 mg/dl (9.4 mmol/l) 4 hours after injection ($P < 0.05$). This effect was maintained at 6 and 8 hours after injection (176 mg/dl [9.87 mmol/l] and 172 mg/dl [9.6 mmol/l], respectively, $P < 0.05$ compared with baseline). In the patients with type 2 diabetes, there was no significant decline in blood glucose from baseline. However, glucose was different from that of the control group at 1 and 6 hours ($P < 0.05$).[89]

Summary

The evidence for bitter melon has come from mostly small studies with weak study design. One small trial indicated that bitter melon may decrease A1C after 7 weeks of use,[90] but there are no long-term trials. Although some patients may benefit from using bitter melon, it may cause low blood glucose when combined with traditional diabetes medications. It should be used with caution by young women of childbearing age, since it may induce menstruation and inadvertently cause miscarriage. There is no information regarding use in lactating women, so it should be avoided in this population. Children should not use bitter melon, since serious adverse effects have occurred, including hypoglycemic coma. Individuals of Mediterranean or Middle-Eastern descent with known G6PDH deficiency or those who have allergies to the melon family should also avoid use. There is no traditional dose, since different forms have been used, including juice, powder, vegetable pulp suspensions, and injectable forms. One source indicated that the dose would be 1 small unripe melon eaten daily or 50–100 ml fresh juice drunk daily with food.[85] However, tinctures and oral supplements are emerging as available sources. Overall bitter melon may be considered safe when eaten as a vegetable, but it is not consistently safe when used in supplement form.

ASIAN GINSENG (*Panax ginseng* C.A. Meyer) AND AMERICAN GINSENG (*Panax quinquefolius* L.)

Ginseng is a botanical product that has been used for medicinal purposes for centuries. Two different forms have been used for diabetes, Asian ginseng (*Panax ginseng* C.A. Meyer) and American ginseng (*P. quinquefolius* L.).[91, 92] The part used is the root.[91]

Both ginseng species are used as an "adaptogen" to deal with stress and to increase energy. Both species are also used in cosmetics and as flavoring ingredients. Although both Asian and American ginsengs have been used as sports performance enhancers, or "ergogenic aids" to help improve physical and athletic stamina, studies do not support this use. Asian ginseng has been used to enhance thinking and memory, to prevent cold or flu, and to prevent cancer. In a double-blind crossover trial, Korean red ginseng improved erectile dysfunction, a malady often found in men with diabetes.[93]

Chemical Constituents and Mechanism of Action

Ginseng contains many different chemical ingredients, but the most active ingredients are a family of steroidal saponins called ginsenosides. Some ginsenosides have opposing effects. For example, ginsenoside Rg1 has hypertensive and central nervous system–stimulant effects, while ginsenoside Rb1 has hypotensive and central nervous system–depressant effects.[75, 94] Some ginsenosides inhibit platelets and have analgesic and anti-inflammatory effects. Both Asian and American ginseng may boost the immune system.[91, 92] Although it is unknown how ginseng may benefit diabetes, animal research has shown that it may decrease the rate of carbohydrate absorption into the portal circulation,[95] increase glucose transport and uptake,[96] and modulate insulin secretion.[97] American ginseng may help decrease postprandial glucose levels.[92, 98]

Adverse Effects and Drug Interactions

Major side effects of ginseng include insomnia and restlessness. Worrisome side effects include increased blood pressure or heart rate. Headache is common, and ginseng may also cause mastalgia, mood changes, and nervousness. Ginseng is unsafe in infants and children, and may not be safe in pregnancy.[91]

Ginseng has been shown to decrease the effectiveness of the blood thinner warfarin (Coumadin),[18] and protection against thromboembolic events is lost. Ginseng decreases the effects of diuretics and hypertension medications.[19] In combination with certain antidepressants, ginseng has resulted in mania.[19] With estrogens, ginseng may produce additive estrogenic effects.[19] Ginseng may inhibit cytochrome P450 (CYP450) 2D6 isoenzymes involved in metabolism of drugs and result in increased effects of drugs such as certain analgesics and some antidepressants.[19] When combined with insulin, sulfonylureas, or other secretagogues, ginseng may cause hypoglycemia.[91]

Clinical Studies

Ginseng has been frequently studied for physical performance or cognitive function as well as immune system effects, but there are few trials where it has been evaluated for diabetes. In one randomized, double-blind study of Asian ginseng in 36 newly diagnosed patients with type 2 diabetes, 12 people each were assigned to placebo, 100 mg/day, or 200 mg/day. Although baseline values were not reported, at the end of the 8-week study, fasting glucose for the three groups was 149 mg/dl (8.3 mmol/l), 139 mg/dl (7.7 mmol/l), and 133 mg/dl (7.4 mmol/l), respectively. (Results were significant only for the 100 mg/day group, $P < 0.05$.) Baseline values were not reported, and the average A1C levels at the end of the study were 6.5, 6.5, and 6%, respectively, for the three groups ($P < 0.05$ for the 200-mg group only).[99] The accuracy of the diagnosis of diabetes or problems with study design may have been an issue.

American ginseng has been studied in people with and without type 2 diabetes. In a small study, subjects with and without diabetes were given a 25-g OGTT, with 3 g ginseng or placebo.[92] Ginseng was given right before or 40 minutes before the OGTT. In subjects without diabetes, there was no difference in postprandial glucose when ginseng was taken right before the OGTT, but when it was taken 40 minutes before, there was a significant decrease in postprandial glucose ($P < 0.05$ vs. placebo). In the participants with diabetes, postprandial glucose decreased whether ginseng was given right before or 40 minutes before the OGTT. The same group of researchers tried the same and higher doses of American ginseng: 3, 6, or 9 g ginseng versus placebo. Glucose decreased in all groups, and there was no difference in effect between the 3-, 6-, and 9-g doses of ginseng.[98]

Summary

Ginseng is available in a variety of forms ranging from cosmetic ingredients to fresh or dried roots to solutions, sodas, and teas.[19] Patients should be aware that there are different types of ginseng but two main types used for diabetes (Asian and American) and that the dose may vary. Both ginseng types have only been studied in type 2 diabetes. There may be inconsistencies in the manufacturing process. One study found that the amount of ginseng stated on the label did not reflect what was contained in the bottle; the ginseng content varied from less (12%) to more (137%) than was indicated on the bottle.[100] Different products have been found to contain other substances, including mandrake root or phenylbutazone, and in one case, an athlete tested positive in a doping test.[101] Ginseng may be safe if taken for 3 months or less. The most common side effect is insomnia, although some people may experience anxiety, headache, and increased blood pressure. It should not be used in children or in pregnant or lactating women. There are many potential drug interactions, so this is a product that should be used with caution when taking other medications. The dose of Asian ginseng is 200 mg daily.[99] The dose of American ginseng is 3 g right before or up to 2 hours before a meal.[92, 98]

NOPAL (*Opuntia streptacantha*)

Nopal is a member of the cactus family and is also known as prickly pear. There are multiple species known as *Opuntia*, including *O. megacantha*, *O. ficus indica*, and *O. streptacantha* Lemaire. Research has focused on *O. streptacantha* Lemaire for its role in lowering blood glucose. Nopal has been used as a food in Mexico and the Southwestern part of the U.S. The leaves, flowers, stems, or fruit are used. Broiled stems or extracts of nopal have been used medicinally to lower blood glucose.[19, 75] Some individuals have prepared blended shakes mixed with fruit.

Nopal has been used to treat diabetes and high cholesterol.[19, 75] One extract has been used to reduce symptoms of hangover.[102] Male patients have also used nopal to reduce symptoms of bladder fullness or urgency (benign prostatic hyperplasia, or BPH).[103]

Chemical Constituents and Mechanism of Action

Nopal contains mucopolysaccharide soluble fibers and phytochemicals, including pectin,[75] which may slow carbohydrate absorption and decrease lipid absorption in the digestive tract. The benefit of nopal does not seem to depend on insulin presence, since it has demonstrated hypoglycemic activity in pancreatectomized animals.[104] An additional theorized mechanism of action is increased insulin sensitivity, since insulin concentrations decrease with nopal administration.[105]

Adverse Effects and Drug Interactions

The major side effects of nopal include mild diarrhea, nausea, abdominal fullness, and increased stool volume.[19, 75] A case report of nopal and chlorpropamide coadministration resulted in additive effects on blood glucose and insulin levels, although hypoglycemia was not reported.[106]

Clinical Studies

Trials studying nopal are small and have mostly been published in Spanish, although abstracts are available in English. One trial was done in three groups of type 2 diabetes patients treated with diet alone or in combination with sulfonylureas.[107] Oral medications were discontinued 72 hours before nopal was administered. After a 12-hour fast, one group of 16 patients received 500 g broiled nopal, a second group of 10 received 400 ml water, and a third group of 6 received 500 g broiled zucchini. Subjects had blood drawn at 60, 120, and 180 minutes after receiving the nopal, water, or zucchini. The nopal group had a significant decline from 222 mg/dl (12.3 mmol/l) fasting to 203 mg/dl (11.3 mmol/l), 198 mg/dl (11.0 mmol/l), and 183 mg/dl (10.2 mmol/l), respectively, at 60, 120, and 180 minutes after receiving the treatment ($P < 0.001$ compared with baseline).[107]

Another trial compared the effects of nopal in 14 patients on sulfonylureas to the effects in individuals without diabetes. Individuals in both groups received 500 g broiled nopal or 400 ml water. In the diabetes group, glucose declined by 21 mg/dl (1.2 mmol/l), 28 mg/dl (1.6 mmol/l), and 41 mg/dl (2.3 mmol/l) at 60, 120, and 180 minutes after nopal was administered ($P < 0.005$ for 60 and 120 minutes vs. baseline;

$P < 0.001$ for 180 minutes vs. baseline).[108] Insulin concentrations also declined significantly.

Summary

Nopal may help lower blood glucose when eaten cooked or taken as a dietary supplement. Although some individuals may prepare a blended shake using raw nopal, the raw stems may not lower blood glucose as effectively as when cooked. Nopal contains fiber and pectin, which may decrease carbohydrate absorption. The major side effects are diarrhea and increased stool volume. There are no long-term studies evaluating nopal for diabetes treatment. It is a benign agent and has been frequently consumed as a food. A frequently quoted dose is 100–500 g daily of broiled stems.[19] An extract containing 1,500 IU taken prior to drinking large quantities of alcohol decreased hangover symptoms.[102] For BPH, the dose used was 500 mg of powdered nopal flowers three times a day.[103] Optimal doses of extracts have not been established to treat diabetes; therefore caution should be exercised regarding recommendation of nopal supplements. As a food, however, it appears quite safe.

ALOE (*Aloe Vera L.*)

Aloe is a member of the Liliaceae family. Derived from the Arabic *alloeh*, the name means "bitter and shiny substance." Aloe grows well in Africa, the Mediterranean, the Caribbean, and warm areas of North and South America. Pictorial wall carvings of aloe have been found in Egyptian temples, and the Egyptian Book of Remedies (circa 1500 B.C.) notes the use of aloe to treat the skin and prepare drugs used as laxatives.[75] Dried aloe leaf juice has been used as a laxative, whereas topical aloe gels have been used to treat wounds, psoriasis, sebhorrhea, sunburn, and dry skin. Orally, aloe has also been used to enhance the immune system and treat diabetes and hyperlipidemia.[75] Aloe is highly used by Hispanic patients and may be called *sábila*.

Chemical Constituents and Mechanism of Action

Two forms of aloe are dried leaf juice and aloe gel.[75] Latex from the pericyclic cells obtained beneath the skin of leaves may be evaporated to form a sticky substance known as "drug aloes" or "aloe." This aloe juice contains cathartics including anthraquinone, barbaloin, a glucoside of aloe-emodin, and other substances. Aloe gel, however, is the ingredient relevant to diabetes. It comes from the inner portion of leaves and does not contain cathartics, but it does contain the polysaccharide glucomannan, which is similar to guar gum.[75] Active ingredients include polysaccharides and glycoprotein, but although the definitive mechanism of action is unknown, the high fiber content alone may promote glucose uptake.[109]

Adverse Effects and Drug Interactions

No adverse effects have been reported with aloe gel. One study evaluated renal and hepatic function, and there were no adverse effects.[110] Aloe did not cause blood glucose to be excessively lowered when combined with the sulfonylurea glibenclamide (glyburide).[110] Nevertheless, caution should be exercised by patients combining aloe with secretagogues. An unusual adverse effect was reported in a case of an individual taking aloe who experienced excessive intraoperative blood loss during surgery where sevoflurane was used. This may be due to the fact that both sevoflurane and aloe inhibit thromboxane A2, which may decrease platelet aggregation and prolong bleeding time.[111] There is also concern that inadvertent inclusion of aloe juice would produce a laxative effect and result in fluid or electrolyte disturbances.

Clinical Studies

In one very small uncontrolled study, five patients with type 2 diabetes were administered one-half teaspoonful dried aloe sap twice daily for 4–14 weeks.[112] Information regarding blinding was not provided. Fasting glucose decreased from a mean 273 mg/dl (15.2 mmol/l) to 151 mg/dl (8.4 mmol/l; $P < 0.001$). Mean A1C also decreased from 10.6% to 8.2% (P value not reported).

A 6-week single-blind, placebo-controlled study was done in 40 patients with newly diagnosed type 2 diabetes.[109] Aloe vera juice was prepared from aloe gel. The patients received 1 tablespoonful aloe gel twice daily or placebo for 6 weeks. Fasting blood measurements were taken weekly, and triglyceride and cholesterol levels were measured every 2 weeks. Fasting glucose declined significantly from 250 mg/dl (13.9 mmol/l) at baseline to 142 mg/dl (7.9 mmol/l) after 6 weeks in the aloe group ($P = 0.01$). Total cholesterol remained unchanged, but triglycerides declined from 220 mg/dl (2.5 mmol/l) to 123 mg/dl (1.4 mmol/l; $P = 0.01$).

Another 6-week single blind controlled trial in 40 patients with type 2 diabetes evaluated the addition of 1 tablespoonful aloe gel or placebo twice daily to the sulfonylurea glibenclamide, 5 mg twice daily.[110] Fasting glucose declined significantly from 288 mg/dl (16.0 mmol/l) to 148 mg/dl (8.2 mmol/l; $P = 0.01$ vs. control) in the aloe vera group. Total cholesterol remained the same: 230 mg/dl (5.95 mmol/l) at baseline and 226 mg/dl (5.80 mmol/l) after 6 weeks. However, triglycerides declined significantly from 265 mg/dl (3.0 mmol/l) to 128 mg/dl (1.5 mmol/l; $P = 0.01$ vs. control).

Summary

Aloe is a tropical plant used to treat type 2 diabetes. The active ingredients are thought to work as fiber to help stimulate cell glucose uptake. No adverse effects have been reported. However, there is concern that additive hypoglycemia may occur if aloe is combined with diabetes drugs. Also, there is a potential for prolonged bleeding with the anesthetic agent sevoflurane during surgery; thus aloe use should be discontinued 2 weeks before surgery. Three small studies have indicated that aloe may decrease fasting glucose and triglycerides, but not total cholesterol. No long-term information regarding aloe use is available, and the effect on A1C was reported in only one very small trial. The dose used has been 1 table-spoonful (15 ml) twice daily of aloe leaf gel.[109, 110] Use of this supplement is not recommended because of the possibility of inadvertent contamination with some of the cathartic ingredients.

BANABA (*Lagerstroemia speciosa* L.)

Banaba is a type of crape myrtle that grows in the Philippines, India, Malaysia, and Australia.[113] Banaba is also known as queen's crape myrtle, queen's flower, and pride of India.[75] The tree is deciduous and has leathery leaves that turn red-orange in the fall. The tree has flowers that are a bright pink to purple and give way to nut-like fruits.[75] It has been used as a folk medicine in the Philippines, and a tea made from the leaves is used to treat diabetes.[113] Other uses include purgative and diuretic actions from the leaf; and root constituents are used for stomach upset.[75] Recently, banaba has become popular in the U.S. It has been used for diabetes and weight loss, although information regarding long-term human use is not available. Information on weight loss is theorized from animal research because of effects on adipocyte differentiation.[75]

Chemical Constituents and Mechanism of Action

Active ingredients include corsolic acid and tannins, including the ellagitannin lagerstroemin. Besides ellagitannins and lagerstroemin, flosin B and reginin A are thought to be glucose-transport enhancers.[114] The ellagitannins are plant polyphenols, which reportedly bind to several polypeptides such as the regulatory subunit of protein kinase A. The active ingredients are thought to stimulate glucose uptake and have insulin-like activity. The latter activity is thought to be secondary to activation of insulin receptor tyrosine kinase or the inhibition of tyrosine phosphatase. Activation of tyrosine kinase causes tyrosine phosphorylation of several proteins, which then induce the functional change of signaling molecules such as phosphatidylinositol 3-kinase.[115] Animal research has shown that banaba may inhibit alpha-amylase and alpha-glucosidases and thus potentially lower elevated postprandial glucose.[75]

Adverse Effects and Drug Interactions

No adverse effects have been reported. Theoretically, banaba may cause blood glucose to be excessively lowered when combined with drugs that can cause hypoglycemia, such as sulfonylureas, or with CAM supplements that have hypoglycemic activity (*Gymnema sylvestre*, American ginseng, etc.). Doses of these medications or CAM supplements may have to be adjusted to prevent excessive lowering of blood glucose.

Clinical Studies

A 15-day randomized control trial was done in 10 patients with type 2 diabetes and fasting glucose levels between 140 mg/dl (7.8 mmol/l) and 250 mg/dl (13.9 mmol/l).[113] Diabetes medications were stopped for 45 days prior to the study. The authors used a 1% corsolic acid extract called Glucosol. Three different doses of banaba—16, 32, or 48 mg—in either a soft gel or hard gel formulation were used. Five subjects in each group received the three different doses for 15 days, with a 10-day washout between doses. Basal glucose was determined by a fasting blood sample 7 days before starting treatment. During the study, three samples were taken, and an average of the three readings was compared to the basal value. The 32- and 48-mg soft gel formulations showed 11% and 30% decrease, respectively, from basal blood glucose values after 15 days of treatment ($P \leq 0.01$ and $P \leq 0.002$, respectively). Only the 48-mg hard gel formulation showed a significant decrease of 20% ($P \leq 0.001$), but the effect was still less than that of the soft gel formulation.

Summary

Banaba is a tropical plant that shows potential benefit to treat type 2 diabetes. It is also being used in multi-ingredient products for weight loss. The active ingredients are thought to stimulate cell glucose uptake by insulin-like activity. In one small study there were no adverse effects or drug interactions reported. This study indicated that banaba may be helpful in lowering blood glucose in patients with type 2 diabetes. However, the authors only reported percentage lowering of blood glucose and did not report the actual values. There is no long-term information available, and the effect on A1C has not been reported. The usual dose is 48 mg/day of the 1% corsolic acid extract, using the soft gel formulation.[113]

CAIAPO (*Ipomoea batatas*)

Caiapo is a form of white sweet potato cultivated in a mountainous region of Kagawa Prefecture, Japan. An extract of the skin of the root has been used as a nutraceutical for type 2 diabetes in Japan.[116] Caiapo has been eaten raw because of the belief that it may help diabetes, hypertension, and anemia. Caiapo also grows in the mountains of South America, and it has also been used by Native Americans to decrease "thirst and weight loss," possible symptoms of diabetes.[117]

Chemical Constituents and Mechanism of Action

An acidic glycoprotein has been isolated from caiapo and is thought to be the active ingredient.[117, 118] The mechanism of action is thought to be improved insulin sensitivity and decreased insulin resistance.

Adverse Effects and Drug Interactions

Adverse effects noted in human studies are mostly gastrointestinal in nature and include constipation, gastrointestinal pain, and meteorism.[116] In theory, caiapo may cause additive hypoglycemia if used with secretagogues or CAM supplements that lower blood glucose.

Clinical Studies

A 6-week pilot study of 18 patients with type 2 diabetes compared 2 g and 4 g caiapo to placebo.[119] Fasting glucose decreased from 158 mg/dl (8.8 mmol/l) to 151 mg/dl (8.4 mmol/l) with low-dose caiapo and from 149 mg/dl (8.3 mmol/l) to 130 mg/dl (7.2 mmol/l) with the higher dose ($P < 0.05$ vs. baseline for the higher dose). The lower dose resulted in unchanged A1C, but A1C decreased from 7.1% to 6.8% with the higher dose (P value not significant). Total and LDL cholesterol also decreased in patients on the higher dose (from 192 mg/dl [5.0 mmol/l] to 172 mg/dl [4.4 mmol/l], $P < 0.05$; and 120 mg/dl [3.1 mmol/l] to 105 mg/dl [2.7 mmol/l], $P < 0.05$, respectively).

Another 3-month randomized, double-blind, placebo-controlled trial was conducted in 61 patients with type 2 diabetes who were mostly diet-treated.[116] Thirty were placed on 4 g/day of caiapo, and 31 were placed on placebo. A1C declined from 7.2% to 6.7% ($P < 0.001$) in those taking caiapo, but increased from 7.04 % at baseline to 7.1% in the placebo group. Fasting glucose declined from 144 mg/dl (8.0 mmol/l) to 129 mg/dl (7.2 mmol/l; $P < 0.001$), and 2-hour postprandial glucose declined from 193 mg/dl (10.7 mmol/l) to 163 mg/dl (9.1 mmol/l; $P < 0.001$). Mean cholesterol was significantly lower in the caiapo group than in the placebo group (215 mg/dl [5.6 mmol/l] vs. 249 mg/dl [6.4 mmol/l], $P < 0.05$). Weight also decreased by 3.7 kg in the caiapo group ($P < 0.0001$ vs. baseline) after 3 months. Blood pressure was unchanged.

Summary

Caiapo is an extract from the root of white-skinned sweet potatoes. There is preliminary information from a small study that 4 g taken once a day before breakfast may help treat type 2 diabetes. It also lowered elevated lipids and produced significant weight loss. Information regarding long-term human use is not available. There are no reports of its use in type 1 diabetes. Adverse effects are mostly gastrointestinal in nature. The dose of caiapo is 4 g/day, based on the randomized controlled trial in type 2 diabetes.[116] It is important to check blood glucose frequently to make sure that it is not lowered excessively. Three months should be allowed to see whether there is an effect on A1C. Caiapo appears to be a potentially useful product, but it is not yet well-known in the U.S.

IVY GOURD (*Coccinia indica*)

Ivy gourd is a unique tropical member of the family Cucurbitaceae.[120] It grows well in India, Southeast Asia, and the Philippines. It has spread to Australia and has been found in Fiji, Tonga, and Hawaii. It is an aggressive climbing perennial vine that spreads quickly over trees and shrubs. The leaves range from 5 to 10 cm (about 2–4 inches) in length and have five lobes that vary from a heart to a pentagon shape. Ivy gourd is a dioecious plant, and the white male and female flowers grow separately. The fruit starts out green and turns red when ripe. Ivy gourd has been classified as a medicinal herb in the traditional practice of ancient Thai medicine. For medicinal purposes, several parts of the plant have been used, including the leaves, roots, stems, and whole plant. The juice of the roots and leaves is used in diabetes, and the leaves are also used as a poultice for skin eruptions.

In Thailand, the young leaves and tips are blanched and prepared in stir-fry dishes, or the leaves are used in curries or for dipping chili paste. Leaves and stems are also added to soup dishes with different meats or noodles. The young leaves are boiled with porridge and then crushed and fed to young children. Other parts of the plant are also used for burns, insect bites, fever, gastrointestinal complaints, and various eye infections.[120]

Chemical Constituents and Mechanism of Action

Ivy gourd contains beta-carotene, a major vitamin A precursor from plant sources.[120] As a food, it is thought to be a good source of protein and fiber, and it contains modest amounts of calcium. However, as a medicinal agent in diabetes, the active ingredients are unknown, although it does contain trace amounts of alkaloids.[121] A quaternary base has been isolated that shows hypoglycemic activity in animal studies. It is thought to suppress the activity of certain enzymes involved in glucose production, such as glucose-6-phosphatase.[122] It is also thought to have some insulin-like activity.[121]

Adverse Effects and Drug Interactions

In the limited number of trials evaluating ivy gourd in diabetes, there have been no side effects reported. A theoretical side effect may be an allergic reaction to some component of the plant. There are no reported cases of drug interactions. In theory, interactions would include possible hypoglycemia when combined with secretagogues or with insulin.

Clinical Studies

A double-blind randomized placebo-controlled trial was conducted in India in 32 patients with type 2 diabetes. Many of the patients were newly diagnosed.[121] Crushed leaf powder was compounded into 300-mg tablets, and 16 patients were randomized to ivy gourd, 16 to placebo. Subjects were asked to take three tablets of the 300-mg leaf extract or three tablets of placebo twice daily for 6 weeks. Subjects were asked not to take any other medications during the study. In the ivy gourd group, two had been treated with sulfonylureas previously, and one with insulin. In the placebo group, four had been treated with sulfonylureas in the past. Subjects were continued on the same diet as before entering the trial. The researchers measured baseline fasting glucose and then administered a 50-g OGTT. Fasting glucose was repeated weekly, and the OGTT was repeated at 6 weeks. Ten of the 16 in the ivy gourd group showed significant improvement in OGTT, whereas no one in the placebo group showed marked improvement. Mean baseline fasting glucose decreased from 179 mg/dl (9.9 mmol/l) at baseline to 122 mg/dl (6.8 mmol/l) at

6 weeks in the ivy gourd group ($P < 0.01$). In the placebo group, mean fasting glucose declined from 195 mg/dl (10.8 mmol/l) at baseline to 181 mg/dl (10.0 mmol/l) at 6 weeks (P value not significant). The 1- and 2-hour OGTT values declined significantly from 268 mg/dl (14.9 mmol/l) and 245 mg/dl (13.6 mmol/l), respectively, at baseline to 225 mg/dl (12.5 mmol/l) and 187 mg/dl (10.4 mmol/l), respectively, at 6 weeks in the ivy gourd group ($P < 0.05$ and $P < 0.01$, respectively). However, the 1- and 2-hour OGTT values were unchanged in the placebo group. The researchers reported there were no side effects and noted no adverse effects on hepatic or kidney function.

Another three-arm controlled trial followed 70 patients with type 2 diabetes for 12 weeks. One group was given 6 g/day dried pellets made from fresh ivy gourd leaves; one group was given sulfonylureas; and one group was given placebo.[123] The open-label design of this study was not as optimal as the design of the previous study. Researchers measured fasting and postprandial glucose. The declines in fasting blood glucose and the OGTT results for those on ivy gourd were similar to the results in those on the sulfonylurea. Fasting glucose declined from 160 mg/dl (8.9 mmol/l) to 110 mg/dl (6.11 mmol/l) after 12 weeks in the ivy gourd group ($P < 0.001$ vs. baseline) and from 165 mg/dl (9.2 mmol/l) to 120 mg/dl (6.7 mmol/l) in the sulfonylurea group (P not significant). There were no side effects reported.

Summary

Ivy gourd is a plant that grows well in India and other tropical areas. It is widely eaten as a vegetable and even fed to young children, and the leaves and root juice are used to treat diabetes or digestive disorders. The active ingredients are unknown, and it has not been studied well in Western medicine. However, in trials conducted in India in type 2 diabetes, it has been shown to decrease fasting and postprandial glucose. No adverse side effects or drug interactions have been reported. The dose used in the trial with better study design was 900-mg, in tablets containing 300-mg ground leaves, taken twice daily.[121] This agent warrants further study, but at this point there is limited evidence for its efficacy in treatment of diabetes. Despite growing interest, it is not yet easily found in the U.S.

HOLY BASIL (*Ocimum sanctum*)

Holy basil is an herb native to India and is regarded as one of the most important plants used in Ayurvedic medicine. It is known by other names, including sacred basil, green holy basil, and hot basil because of the peppery taste.[19] Another name is *tulsi*, a Hindu word meaning "the incomparable one." It has a pleasant aroma and is available in both red and green varieties. It is planted and grows abundantly around Hindu temples,[19] and although it is native to India, it is now widely grown throughout the world. The plant is hairy with multiple branches with small, tender leaves. The leaves, stems, seeds, and oil are used medicinally, but it is a common ingredient in Indian cuisine in soups and stir-fry dishes.[19]

Although holy basil has been used to treat diabetes, it has primarily been used to treat common colds, influenza, asthma, malaria, and tuberculosis.[19, 124] It has been used as a mosquito repellant and a topical treatment for ringworm. It has also been used as an antidote for scorpion and snake bites.[19] In animals it has analgesic and fever-reducing properties and protective effects against the ulcer-producing effects of anti-inflammatory drugs such as aspirin.[125, 126] Another popular use is for stress.[19]

Chemical Constituents and Mechanism of Action

The leaves contain essential oils that yield eugenol, methyl eugenol, and caryophyllene but also other substances such as ursolic acid and apigenin.[127] Other ingredients include the monoterpenes (camphor, cineol, geraniol, and ocimene), sesquiterpenes, and phenylpropanes (methyl cinnamate).[124] Active constituents are thought to be eugenol, linalool, and methyl chavicol (or estragole).[124] It is unknown which of the chemical components may be responsible for the benefit in diabetes. Researchers have theorized that holy basil leaves may improve pancreatic β-cell function and thus enhance insulin secretion.[127]

Adverse Effects and Drug Interactions

In the one major trial for diabetes in humans, no side effects were reported. However, in animals, holy basil may decrease sperm count and thus possibly decrease fertility.[128, 129]

There are no reported cases of drug interactions involving holy basil. Theoretical interactions would be possible hypoglycemia when combined with secretagogues or insulin. In animals, one component, holy basil seed oil, may increase risk of bleeding;[130] thus caution is warranted if combined with antiplatelet drugs such as aspirin, warfarin, clopidogrel, or CAM supplements that have antiplatelet activity. In theory, holy basil may also interact with sedatives from the phenobarbital family, since in an animal study there was an increased pentobarbitone-induced duration of sleep.[130]

Clinical Studies

There is only one small controlled trial in 40 patients with type 2 diabetes.[127] Half the patients had well-established type 2 diabetes and were on oral diabetes medications. Patients were asked to stop their diabetes medications 7 days before the start of the trial; then all patients were given a holy basil leaf extract for a run-in period of 5 days. Half were randomly assigned to take 2.5 g holy basil leaf powder and 20 were given placebo for 4 weeks and then crossed over to the other treatment group without a washout period for another 4 weeks. Researchers measured fasting and 2-hour postprandial blood glucose as well as total cholesterol. In the first group, mean fasting glucose declined from 134.5 mg/dl (7.5 mmol/l) to 99.7 mg/dl (5.5 mmol/l) after 4 weeks of treatment with holy basil. After patients crossed over to placebo for 4 weeks, fasting glucose increased to 115.6 mg/dl (6.4 mmol/l). In the placebo-first group, mean fasting glucose declined from 132.4 mg/dl (7.4 mmol/l) to 123.2 mg/dl (6.8 mmol/l) after 4 weeks and then declined even further to 97.2 mg/dl (5.4 mmol/l) after they crossed over to holy basil for 4 weeks. Overall, mean fasting blood glucose was 21 mg/dl (1.2 mmol/l) lower in the holy basil group. Postprandial blood glucose decreased during the 4-week treatment with holy basil from 223.9 mg/dl (12.4 mmol/l) to 204 mg/dl (11.3 mmol/l), and total cholesterol decreased from 238.2 mg/dl (6.2 mmol/l) to 221.5 mg/dl (5.7 mmol/l). However, the results were not significant. There were no adverse effects reported by those taking holy basil or placebo.

Summary

Holy basil is an important herb used in Ayurvedic medicine. It is used for a variety of ailments such as respiratory disorders, arthritis, and inflammation, as well as stress and diabetes. In type 2 diabetes patients, a leaf extract was found to reduce fasting blood glucose by 17.6% and postprandial blood glucose by 7.3% as well as to result in a small decrease in total cholesterol. Although it has been widely studied in animals, there is only one small trial reported in humans with type 2 diabetes. No adverse side effects have been reported in humans, but the longest it has been studied is 4 weeks. Caution is warranted because animal data indicates a potential for bleeding reactions if combined with antiplatelet drugs or herbs (ginkgo, garlic, ginger, or others) and a possibility of lowered sperm count. There is no typical dose, but in one study, 2.5 g dried leaf powder was used once a day on an empty stomach.[127] This is one of the many products that is probably appropriate in diabetes when used as a food, but questionable in an actual supplement form.

VIJAYASAR (*Pterocarpus marsupium* Roxb. [Leguminoceae])

Vijayasar is also known as the Indian kino tree. It is a large deciduous tree found in central India and Sri Lanka. It is used as a traditional Indian medicine for diabetes, and research on its hypoglycemic activity has mostly been conducted in animals with experimentally induced diabetes.[131–133] An aqueous or ethanol extract of the bark or wood may be used.[132]

Chemical Constituents and Mechanism of Action

The active ingredients are (–)epicatechin, a benzopyran, and phenolic constituents including marsupsin, ptorosupin, and pterostilbene.[131, 134] The mechanism of action is thought to be related to increased islet cyclic adenosine monophosphate content, which may increase insulin release. Other actions are to facilitate conversion of proinsulin (C-peptide) to insulin and to produce insulin-like effects.[131, 134]

Adverse Effects and Drug Interactions

There are no adverse effects reported. One study evaluated effects of Vijayasar on electrolytes (hepatic, renal, and hematological function) and weight and did not report any harmful effects in the patients.[134] In theory, additive hypoglycemia may occur if Vijayasar is used in combination with secretagogues or CAM supplements that decrease blood glucose.

Clinical Studies

There are a few short-term studies in small numbers of patients where a slight benefit has been found with use of Vijayasar. A 12-week open-label study in 97 patients with newly diagnosed type 2 diabetes reported benefit with Vijayasar.[134] In this study, patients were placed on medical nutrition therapy for 1 month, consuming a diet consisting of 60–65% carbohydrate, 10–15% protein, and 25–30% fat. Those patients who had fasting glucose of 120–180 mg/dl (6.7–10.0 mmol/l) and postprandial values of 180–250 mg/dl (10.0–13.9 mmol/l) were then treated with twice daily doses of Vijayasar at a starting dose of 2 g/day. At the end of 4 weeks, patients with fasting glucose or postprandial glucose higher than target values (fasting $\geq$120 mg/dl [6.7 mmol/l] or postprandial $\geq$180 mg/dl [10.0 mmol/l]) were treated with 3 g/day. At the end of 4 more weeks, those individuals with higher-than-target fasting or postprandial values were then treated with 3 g/day. Fasting glucose values declined from a mean baseline of 151 mg/dl (8.4 mmol/l) to 119 mg/dl

(6.6 mmol/l) at 12 weeks ($P < 0.001$). Mean postprandial glucose values decreased from the mean baseline of 216 mg/dl (12 mmol/l) to 171 mg/dl (9.5 mmol/l; $P < 0.001$). Mean baseline A1C decreased from 9.8% to 9.4% ($P < 0.001$), and 7% of participants achieved the study's target A1C value of $\leq 8.5\%$. Although lipids were also measured, there was only a nonsignificant decrease in triglycerides.

Summary

Vijayasar is a plant product from the bark of the Indian kino tree.[131] It has a long history of use for diabetes in India, although there is a paucity of studies that evaluate its effectiveness. Overall, Vijayasar has been found in an open-label study to significantly decrease fasting and postprandial glucose in newly diagnosed type 2 diabetes patients.[134] A total of 72% of patients achieved target fasting blood glucose, and 75% achieved target postprandial values. Most patients, 73%, achieved the target values with the 2 g/day dose.[134] Vijayasar is a traditional Indian medicine that is gaining popularity, and although there is preliminary evidence for its benefit, there is insufficient evidence to recommend its use.

JAMBOLAN (*Eugenia jambolana* or *Syzygium cumini*)

Jambolan is also known by a variety of names, including jambul, jamun beej, Java plum, and rose apple.[19, 124] The tree produces edible fruit and is native to India, Sri Lanka, and other parts of Southeast Asia, but it now grows in South America and Florida. It attains a height of 50–100 feet (about 15–30 meters).[124, 135] Jambolan is highly consumed as a tea in Brazil.[136]

Chemical Constituents and Mechanism of Action

The seeds contain gallic and ellagic acid, corilagin, and other active ingredients, including quercetin.[124, 135] Tannins are also thought to contribute pharmacological effects.[19] The overall mechanism of action is not well-known, but in addition to some hypoglycemic effects, the seeds may also possess antihypertensive and anti-inflammatory properties. In mice, decreased activity and other neuropsychopharmacologic effects have been seen.[124]

Adverse Effects and Drug Interactions

Thus far, no adverse effects have been reported, although various clinical parameters have been assessed in a small study.[137] Hepatic, renal, and lipid tests showed no adverse changes from baseline in this small 28-day study. There are no reported drug interactions, although there is the potential for additive hypoglycemia when used concomitantly with insulin or secretagogues. Because of the central nervous system effects seen in animals, there is a theoretical possibility of additive effects with central nervous system depressants.[124]

Clinical Studies

There are only small studies with conflicting results. One positive 3-month study was done in 30 patients with type 2 diabetes who were given 4 g crushed jambolan powder three times a day for 3 months.[138] The patients were compared with six patients on 250 mg/day of the sulfonylurea chlorpropamide. Mean fasting blood glucose decreased significantly at 2 months in the jambolan group, by 52 mg/dl (2.9 mmol/l) from a baseline of 163 mg/dl (9.1 mmol/l; $P < 0.001$). The decrease was not significant at 3 months (32 mg/dl [1.78 mmol/l] from baseline). However, OGTT was significantly lower than baseline both at 2 ($P < 0.001$) and 3 months ($P < 0.01$); the results were not significant when compared with chlorpropamide. The study design was faulty, since patient demographic details were not stated.

A negative trial reported the effects of a comparison among three groups of patients.[137] In this randomized, double-blind, placebo-controlled trial, 27 patients were randomized to the groups after a 3-month run-in period and followed for 28 days. One group was randomized to jambolan tea plus placebo tablets twice daily, another was randomized to placebo tea plus glyburide (5 mg twice daily), and the last group was randomized to placebo tea and placebo tablets twice daily. Patients were asked to drink the tea (placebo or 2 g/day dry leaf in a teabag steeped for 5 minutes in 1 liter water) as a water substitute. Fasting glucose increased significantly from a mean baseline of 157 mg/dl (8.7 mmol/l) to 164 mg/dl (9.1 mmol/l; $P = 0.015$) at 28 days in the jambolan group. In contrast, fasting glucose decreased from mean baseline of 158 mg/dl (8.8 mmol/l) to 122 mg/dl (6.8 mmol/l) in the glyburide group. Fructosamine decreased slightly in both groups, but the decrease was not significant (jambolan, 3.5 mmol/l at baseline and 3.4 mmol/l at 28 days, $P = 0.946$; glyburide, 3.5 mmol/l at baseline and 3.2 mmol/l at 28 days, P value not stated).

Summary

Jambolan is another traditional plant product that has been used in India, Sri Lanka, and South America. The tree grows well in Florida as well, and the fruit is edible. It is consumed as a tea, and studies have shown little to no benefit. Even in animals, there has been no therapeutic benefit. Although there are no reported adverse effects or drug interactions, caution should be exercised because, in theory, hypoglycemia may occur. Jambolan has been included as an ingredient in multi-ingredient dietary supplements used to treat diabetes. At this time there is insufficient evidence of the supplement's benefit as a treatment for diabetes, although jambolan may be consumed as a food.

BLONDE PSYLLIUM (*Plantago ovata*)

Blonde psyllium is also known by several other names, including plantago psyllium, ispaghula husk, or simply psyllium.[19, 139] The plant grows in India, the Middle East, parts of Europe, including Spain and the Canary Islands, and Arizona and Brazil.[140] It bears flowers and fruit, but the relevant part of the plant so far is the seed and seed husk. Although psyllium is primarily used as a bulk-forming laxative and for diarrhea and irritable bowel syndrome, it is also used for hyperlipidemia. In people with diabetes, other uses have been to decrease postprandial glucose and lower cholesterol.[19]

Chemical Constituents and Mechanism of Action

Psyllium is a mixture of acidic and neutral polysaccharides with galacturonic acid. The polysaccharides are composed of monomers of D-xylose and L-arabinose and pentosanes.[139] The mechanism of action is probably similar to that of other soluble fibers or gel-forming substances.[141, 142] It has been theorized that in aqueous solution psyllium forms a viscous gel that slows glucose absorption into the small intestine and thereby allows a decrease in postprandial peak glucose values.[141] Another potential mechanism is a delay in gastric emptying that diminishes postprandial hyperglycemia. Another possible mechanism is carbohydrate sequestering, slowing carbohydrate access to digestive enzymes. Some studies have demonstrated a "second-meal effect," possibly because the soluble fiber may elicit a lower postprandial increase in insulin concentrations with a smaller counterregulatory meal response.[141] The lipid-lowering effects may be due to absorption of dietary fats and decreased systemic absorption. Psyllium may also enhance cholesterol elimination in fecal bile acids.[19]

Adverse Effects and Drug Interactions

Allergic reactions including cough and sinusitis have been reported, as well as adverse gastrointestinal effects, including flatulence.[19, 140] The inner seed parts may be responsible for the allergic reactions.[19] Swallowing disorders may occur due to possible esophageal obstruction.[19] Individuals with phenylketonuria may have problems if the supplement is sweetened with aspartame. Some products contain sugars that may increase blood glucose.

There are a variety of drug interactions, mainly due to binding and thus decreased absorption of medications taken at the same time as psyllium.[19]

This includes decreased carbamazepine, iron supplement, and riboflavin absorption. Additive effects may occur with hypoglycemic drugs as well as lipid-lowering agents. Taking psyllium with orlistat and misoprostol has improved gastrointestinal tolerability of these agents. Additive effects with certain statins and other lipid-lowering agents have led to improved lipid profiles.

Clinical Studies

Several small studies demonstrate the benefit of psyllium in reducing postprandial glucose and lipids. One frequently quoted study had a randomized, placebo-controlled, crossover design in 18 patients with type 2 diabetes.[141] The patients received twice-daily psyllium or placebo before a standardized breakfast and supper in two study phases that were 15 hours each. Glucose was measured at baseline for each phase, and postprandial values were measured every 15 minutes for 2 hours, then once after 30 minutes and hourly thereafter for 2.5 more hours. A 7-day washout was followed by a second test period when patients were crossed over to the opposite group. The authors reported that peak postprandial glucose value elevations were 14% lower than with placebo after breakfast (109 mg/dl [6.0 mmol/l] vs. 126 mg/dl [7.0 mmol/l]) and 21% lower after dinner (54 mg/dl [3.0 mmol/l] vs. 68 mg/dl [3.8 mmol/l]), although these numbers did not achieve statistical significance and the authors did not state specific glucose values. The authors reported that postlunch numbers were reduced even further, by 31%, and it was speculated that this was a "second-meal" or residual effect of the psyllium.

One of the largest studies was a double-blind, placebo-controlled trial in 125 patients with type 2 diabetes who initiated dietary therapy for 6 weeks and then took 5 g psyllium or placebo three times daily for 6 weeks.[142] Mean plasma glucose values declined 6 weeks after diet treatment (values not stated but shown in a graph). After an additional 6 weeks of psyllium, mean plasma glucose declined even further (no values given, only a graph showing that end point values were ~140 mg/dl [7.8 mmol/l] and ~175 mg/dl [9.7 mmol/l] 6 weeks earlier). The authors stated that there was a significant difference between the psyllium group and the placebo group ($P < 0.01$). Mean LDL cholesterol also declined after 6 weeks of psyllium use (141 mg/dl [3.7 mmol/l to 118 mg/dl [3.1 mmol/l], $P < 0.01$).

A randomized, double-blind, placebo-controlled trial assessed 34 men with type 2 diabetes for 10 weeks.[143] Following a 2-week dietary stabilization phase, the patients were randomized to 5.1 g psyllium or placebo twice daily. After psyllium treatment, metabolic-ward serum concentrations showed that all-day mean plasma glucose declined from 214 mg/dl (11.9 mmol/l) to 205 mg/dl (11.4 mmol/l), whereas in the placebo group, glucose increased from 208 mg/dl (11.6 mmol/l) to 222 mg/dl (12.3 mmol/l; an 11% difference between the two, $P < 0.05$). Postlunch concentrations declined from 193 mg/dl (10.7 mmol/l) to 180 mg/dl (10 mmol/l) in the psyllium group and increased from 187 mg/dl (10.4 mmol/l) to 211 mg/dl (11.7 mmol/l) in the placebo group (a 19.2% difference between the two groups, $P = 0.01$). LDL cholesterol decreased by 4.7% in the psyllium group and increased by 8.3% in the placebo group (a 13% difference that was not significant). Total cholesterol decreased by 2.1% in the psyllium group and increased by 6.9% in the placebo group (a significant 9% difference, $P < 0.05$).

Summary

Blonde psyllium is a mainstream product that is available to treat constipation and has been recognized as a cholesterol-lowering agent. A commonly used form is the nonprescription product Metamucil.[144] Although readily available as a nonprescription medication, it has not been approved for its glucose-lowering effects and is therefore considered an empiric supplement for lowering postprandial glucose. People with diabetes should be cautioned to use products that contain sugar substitutes, although those with phenylketonuria should avoid the aspartame-containing products. Although the American Heart Association (AHA) has not included psyllium in a stepwise dietary approach, the FDA has allowed foods containing at least 1.7 g psyllium to claim reduced heart disease risk when ingested as part of a low-fat and low-cholesterol diet.[145] The dose used to lower lipids has been 5.1 g twice daily or 3.4 g three times daily. The dose to lower postprandial glucose has ranged from 5.1 g twice daily to 5.1 g three times daily.

GLUCOMANNAN (*Amorphophallus konjac* K. Koch)

Glucomannan is also known as konjac or konjac mannan. The plant, *Amorphophallus konjac*, is grown in Indonesia and Japan. The plant tubers yield a chemical known as konjac mannan. Konjac flour is treated with cupric hydroxide and washed with ethanol or dialysis against water.[75] In Asia, it has been popular as a medicinal agent and food for thousands of years. Glucomannan is extracted from the tubers, dried, and molded into noodles, rubbery jelly, and other food products.[146] Glucomannan has been used as a bulk-forming laxative, but it has also been used for weight loss, hyperlipidemia, and diabetes.[124]

Chemical Constituents and Mechanism of Action

Glucomannan is a polysaccharide composed of glucose and mannose. It is derived from konjac flour by chemical treatment and ethanol washings.[75] This agent contains soluble fiber that may delay glucose absorption and decrease cholesterol absorption. It is thought to inhibit cholesterol absorption in the jejunum, inhibit bile acid absorption in the ileum, and possibly reduce stimulation of hydro-3-methyl-glutaryl CoA reductase.[147] Another possible lipid-lowering mechanism is increased fecal sterol excretion.[146] Another proposed mechanism is production of short-chain fatty acids that may decrease hepatic synthesis of cholesterol.[147] Effects on blood glucose may be related to increased viscosity and subsequent slowed rate of food absorption in the small intestine.[147, 148]

Adverse Effects and Drug Interactions

The most dangerous adverse effect is esophageal obstruction, which has been reported with the tablet form but not with powders or capsules. It may cause stomach upset. Drug interactions may include binding of oil-soluble vitamins such as A, D, E, and K. Also, there may be additive effects with glucose-lowering agents as well as with antihyperlipidemics.[19, 124]

Clinical Studies

There are a variety of studies using glucomannan in people with diabetes. Most have a small number of subjects. One was a double-blind, placebo-controlled, crossover study in 11 patients receiving treatment for type 2 diabetes, hyperlipidemia, and hypertension.[147] The patients were initially placed on National Cholesterol Education Program (NCEP) Step-2 diet that limited cholesterol and saturated fat intake for 8 weeks. After the diet treatment phase, patients were randomized for 3 weeks to placebo or treatment consisting of konjac biscuits eaten three times a day to provide 0.7 g /100 dietary calories. At the end of 3 weeks, patients had a 2-week washout and were then crossed over to the other group. Mean fructosamine declined 6.1% from mean baseline 3.36 mmol/l (P not significant) in the treatment group and decreased by 0.5% from mean baseline 3.25 mmol/l (P not significant) in the placebo group. However, the treatment difference of 5.7% between groups was significant (P = 0.007). Fasting glucose decreased significantly from a mean baseline of 173 mg/dl (9.63 mmol/l) to 154 mg/dl (8.6 mmol/l; P = 0.004) in the konjac group, whereas it decreased nonsignificantly by 1.5% from 167 mg/dl (9.3 mmol/l) in the placebo group. Between-treatment difference was not significant. Mean baseline total cholesterol (236 mg/dl [6.1 mmol/l] and 225 mg/dl [5.8 mmol/l], respectively) decreased in both the treatment and the placebo group, by 16% and 5% (P = 0.001 for the treatment group; P not significant for placebo). The 11% between-treatment difference was not significant after Bonferroni-Hochberg correction. Mean baseline

LDL cholesterol decreased significantly from 150 mg/dl (3.9 mmol/l) to 113 mg/dl (2.9 mmol/l) in the treatment group ($P = 0.001$) and from 137 mg/dl (3.6 mmol/l) to 130 mg/dl (3.4 mmol/l; P not significant for placebo). The 19% between-treatment difference was not significant after Bonferroni-Hochberg correction. Systolic pressure decreased significantly by 5.5% in the treatment group ($P = 0.003$) and increased by 1.4% in the placebo group (baseline 139.5 mmHg and 128.8 mmHg, respectively). The between-treatment difference was significant (6.9%, $P = 0.021$). There were no differences in diastolic blood pressure.

Another randomized, double-blind, placebo-controlled trial was done in 22 patients with type 2 diabetes and hyperlipidemia.[146] Patients were on oral diabetes medications but not on antihyperlipidemics. The patients followed an NCEP diet for 2 months, then were randomized to placebo or glucomannan. After 28 days, they were crossed over to the other group without a washout. The dose used was lower than in the previous study, 0.24 g/100 dietary calories vs. 0.7 g/100 calories. LDL cholesterol decreased significantly in the treatment group from baseline of 154 mg/dl (4.0 mmol/l) to 138 mg/dl (3.6 mmol/l; $P = 0.023$), while it increased in the placebo group (150 mg/dl [3.9 mmol/l] at baseline to 165 mg/dl [4.3 mmol/l]). Between-treatment difference was significant, 20.7% ($P = 0.0004$). HDL increased significantly from 44 mg/dl (1.2 mmol/l) to 46 mg/dl (1.3 mmol/l; $P = 0.034$), while there was a nonsignificant drop in HDL in the placebo group (44 mg/dl [1.2 mmol/l], decrease of 0.5%). Between-treatment difference was not significant. Mean fasting glucose declined significantly in the treatment group from 169 mg/dl (9.4 mmol/l) to 148 mg/dl (8.2 mmol/l; $P = 0.002$), and in the placebo group it increased from 157 mg/dl (8.7 mmol/l) to 173 mg/dl (9.6 mmol/l; $P = 0.017$). Between-treatment difference between groups was significant, 23.2% ($P = 0.002$). Mean 2-hour postprandial glucose also declined by 30 mg/dl (1.7 mmol/l) in the treatment group, from 248 mg/dl (13.8 mmol/l; $P = 0.006$), and increased nonsignificantly in the placebo group. Between-treatment difference was not significant for postprandial glucose.

Summary

Glucomannan is a polysaccharide that has been used for hyperlipidemia and hyperglycemia. There are a variety of small randomized, controlled trials that have shown improvement in lipids, fasting and postprandial glucose, and systolic blood pressure. A larger study that used glucomannan in food form for 2 months demonstrated decreased fasting and 2-hour postprandial glucose values as well as a decreased A1C and a 2-kg weight loss.[149] There is no problem with its use as a food, but as a supplement in tablet form, it has caused esophageal obstruction. If glucomannan is to be used, it should be consumed in powder or capsule form. It may cause gastrointestinal upset and may have additive effects with diabetes and lipid-lowering medications. It should not be taken at the same time as oil-soluble vitamins. The dose used has been variable, ranging from 3.6 g/day to 10.6 g/day for diabetes and hyperlipidemia.[19]

GUAR GUM (*Cyamopsis tetragonolobus* [L.] Taub)

The guar plant, or Indian cluster bean, is indigenous to tropical parts of Asia, India, and Pakistan and is also grown in the southern U.S. The small plant bears seed-containing pods. Guar gum is a soluble fiber obtained from the endosperm, which comprises almost half the seed weight. The endosperm is separated from the plant and used to produce the commercial product.[75] Although guar gum has been used as a thickening agent in both medications and foods, it also is used in the textile and oil-drilling industries. Tablets containing a guar gum matrix are being evaluated and used for sustained-release product delivery. Medicinal uses include bulking stool, promoting weight loss, and decreasing pruritus in intrahepatic cholestasis. It has also been used for diabetes and hyperlipidemia.[75]

Chemical Constituents and Mechanism of Action

Like glucomannan, guar gum is a polysaccharide, but it is formed from galactomannan. The food-grade product contains primarily guaran, a galactomannan composed of D-mannose and D-galactose units. When combined with water, it forms a viscous gel varying in pH from neutral to slightly acidic.[75]

The mechanism of the lipid-lowering effect is thought to be decreased cholesterol absorption and increased bile excretion, resulting in increased hepatic cholesterol turnover. The lipid-lowering activity may be similar to bile acid sequestrants. Hypoglycemic effects are thought to be due to altered gastrointestinal transit and delayed glucose absorption. Because it causes a feeling of fullness, guar gum is thought to promote decreased food intake and possibly weight loss.[75]

Adverse Effects and Drug Interactions

The main adverse effects are gastrointestinal upset, including nausea, flatulence, and diarrhea. In weight loss products, guar gum's water-retention properties may result in swelling of the product, leading to esophageal obstruction.[75]

Guar gum may have additive effects with lipid-lowering agents or diabetes medications. Additive effects have been reported when guar gum was coadministered with lovastatin.[150] It may also decrease absorption of drugs that are taken at the same time; this has been reported with metformin, some sulfonylureas, digoxin, and penicillin.[75]

Clinical Studies

Several studies have evaluated guar gum in people with type 1 or type 2 diabetes. One 6-week randomized, double-blind, placebo-controlled study in 17 type 1 diabetes patients evaluated use of 5 g granulated guar gum or placebo four times a day, before meals and as an evening snack.[151] Specifically, mean fasting glucose decreased significantly from 157 mg/dl (8.7 mmol/l) at baseline to 126 mg/dl (7.0 mmol/l) after 6 weeks in the guar gum group ($P < 0.01$) and increased from 139 mg/dl (7.7 mmol/l) to 144 mg/dl (8.0 mmol/l) in the placebo group (not significant). Mean A1C declined significantly from 8.3% to 7.7% in the guar gum group

($P < 0.01$) and from 7.9% to 7.4% in the placebo group (not significant). Mean LDL cholesterol decreased significantly in the guar gum group from baseline of 189 mg/dl (4.9 mmol/l) to 158 mg/dl (4.1 mmol/l) at end point ($P < 0.001$) and increased from baseline of 163 mg/dl (4.2 mmol/l) to 166 mg/dl (4.3 mmol/l) at end point in the placebo group (results not significant). Mean triglyceride and HDL cholesterol values remained unchanged in both groups.

A long-term, randomized, single-blind, placebo-controlled study evaluated guar gum use in 15 people with diet-treated type 2 diabetes for 48 weeks. The patients took 5 g guar gum three times daily with meals.[152] Patients took placebo for 8 weeks, then guar gum for 48 weeks, then placebo again for an additional 8 weeks. Glucose values, postprandial glucose, and lipids improved during treatment with guar gum. Mean A1C during treatment with guar gum was 8.5%, compared with 9% during the first placebo treatment ($P = 0.015$), but remained the same during the second placebo treatment period. Mean fasting glucose was 171 mg/dl (9.5 mmol/l) during the first placebo treatment and 166 mg/dl (9.2 mmol/l) during the guar gum treatment period (results not significant). However, mean fasting glucose rose significantly during the second placebo treatment period (185 mg/dl [10.3 mmol/l], $P = 0.004$ vs. guar gum). Mean LDL cholesterol during the first placebo period decreased from 150 mg/dl (3.9 mmol/l) to 137 mg/dl (3.6 mmol/l) during guar gum treatment ($P = 0.029$) and increased to 166 mg/dl (4.3 mmol/l) during the second placebo period ($P = 0.001$ vs. guar gum). Mean HDL and triglyceride cholesterol values remained unchanged.

Summary

Guar gum is another type of soluble fiber used for treatment of diabetes and hyperlipidemia. For weight loss, guar gum has not been effective.[153] Guar gum has been studied mostly in small numbers of patients, and there are few long-term studies. In one study in type 2 diabetes, however, guar gum improved long-term glucose control as well as LDL cholesterol. Triglycerides and HDL cholesterol values did not improve. Overall, guar gum has been shown to decrease fasting and postprandial glucose as well as lipids, but patients should be told that although this is an agent that may improve diabetes and hyperlipidemia, results are modest.

In one study of 40 patients with diabetes, A1C decreased from high values of 12.6% and 12.0% to 10.5% and 10.9%, respectively, after 3 months, using two different guar gum preparations.[154] Effects were modest, showing that in people with uncontrolled diabetes, guar gum makes only a small difference in A1C and does not achieve target values. Concomitant use of guar gum with diabetes medications and antihyper-lipidemics may result in additive effects, but patients should be counseled that guar gum should not be taken at the same time as other medications because it may impair their absorption. Patients should be warned about the adverse gastrointestinal effects, and A1C and lipid parameters should be monitored closely.

STEVIA (*Stevia rebaudiana* Bertoni)

Stevia is a plant that grows in Paraguay, Brazil, Central America, some Middle Eastern countries, Southeast Asia, and China. There are more than 300 species of this plant, which belongs to the family Asteraceae/Compositae. Stevia is a small, shrubby perennial that bears small white flowers. The applicable part is the leaf.[124]

Stevia has been used as a noncaloric sweetener in South America and Japan for over 20 years.[155] In a comparison of other sweeteners, aspartame is 200 times sweeter than sugar, sucralose is 600 times sweeter, and stevia is 200–300 times sweeter.[156] In some Asian countries, it is used in foods such as soy sauce, pickled products, or dried seafood to diminish the salty taste. It has also been used for diabetes, hypertension, and as a cardiotonic agent.[155, 157] In animals, it has shown contraceptive activity.[19]

Chemical Constituents and Mechanism of Action

Stevia contains diterpene glycosides: stevioside (composed of three glucose units), dulcoside, and rebaudiosides. Stevioside is linked to a diterpenic carboxylic alcohol known as steviol.[124] Steviolbioside is another component.[157] The leaves contain many other chemical constituents as well.

The mechanism of action is very complex. The steviosides and related compounds inhibit oxidative phosphorylation by inhibition of nucleotide exchange, uncoupling of respiration, and inhibition of NADH-oxidase, L-glutamate dehydrogenase, and succinate dehydrogenase. All of these effects may result in an increase in glucose utilization. These compounds may also inhibit gluconeogenesis.[157] Stevioside and steviol have been shown in murine research to directly affect β-cells and result in insulin secretion.[158]

The mechanism for lowering blood pressure is thought to be calcium-channel blockade similar to that of verapamil,[155] but in animals, it also has shown vasodilation and diuretic activity.[19]

Adverse Effects and Drug Interactions

The primary adverse effects have included nausea, bloating, dizziness, headache, asthenia, and myalgia.[155] Because it belongs to the family Asteraceae/Compositae, it may have cross-allergies in people who are allergic to ragweed, marigolds, chrysanthemums, or daisies.[19] In animals, nephrotoxicity and mutagenicity have been reported.[124, 156] In 2-year trials in humans, there were no adverse effects on electrolytes, creatinine, liver function, or lipids.[155] Theoretical drug interactions would include additive hypoglycemia with secretagogues and hypotension if combined with calcium-channel blockers or other antihypertensives.

Clinical Studies

Two small studies address the issue of the impact on blood glucose. One was in normal subjects. The study in 16 subjects without diabetes consisted of a 100-g OGTT given first without stevia and then 21 hours later with stevia administered 2 hours before starting the test.[157] The subjects then received 13 doses, 5 g each, of stevia aqueous extract given at 6-hour intervals. The control group consisted of 6 subjects who received 13 doses of arabinose. Plasma glucose values decreased significantly with stevia administration ($P < 0.01$ for all times except 120 minutes, when $P < 0.05$). The authors did not provide actual numbers, only a figure, and the approximate values at 30 minutes were 128 mg/dl (7.1 mmol/l) without stevia and 103 mg/dl (5.7 mmol/l) with stevia.

A crossover study assessed stevia or placebo given with a test meal in 12 patients with type 2 diabetes.[159] Mean A1C was 7.4%. Patients were given 1 g stevia or maize starch with the meal. Blood was drawn 30 minutes before the meal and at various times for 240 minutes thereafter. Stevia significantly decreased postprandial blood glucose by 18% ($P < 0.004$). Area under the curve glucose value was 522 mmol/l for stevia and 639 mmol/l for maize starch ($P < 0.02$).

Stevia has also been studied in hypertension. A 1-year trial using 250 mg three times a day in people without diabetes showed a significant improvement in systolic (14 mmHg decrease, $P < 0.05$) and diastolic blood pressure (12 mmHg, $P < 0.05$).[160] A 2-year hypertension trial in 162 Chinese subjects with hypertension but without diabetes also showed benefit.[155] In this multicenter, randomized, double-blind, placebo-controlled trial, the subjects took 500 mg stevioside powder or placebo three times a day for 2 years. In the stevia group, mean baseline systolic blood pressure decreased from 150 mmHg at baseline to 140 mmHg at end point ($P < 0.005$). In the placebo group, mean baseline systolic pressure was 149 mmHg at baseline and 150 mmHg at end point. The difference between stevia and placebo was significant ($P < 0.05$). Mean diastolic pressure decreased from 95 mmHg at baseline to 89 mmHg at end point in the stevia group ($P < 0.05$). Mean diastolic pressure decreased from 96 mmHg to 95 mmHg in the placebo group. The difference between groups was significant ($P < 0.05$).

Summary

Stevia is a noncaloric sweetener that has been used in countries such as Brazil and Japan for decades. Although small doses and occasional use may be benign, stevia has not received FDA approval as a sweetener, although it is available as a dietary supplement. There are concerns relating to mutagenicity. Other regulatory bodies, including those of Australia, Canada, and the European Union, as well as the Joint Expert Committee on Food Additives (JECFA), an international scientific group working under the United Nations and the World Health Organization, have chosen not to approve stevia as a food.[156] The JECFA has stated that a daily intake of up to 2 mg/kg of body weight is acceptable, and more data will be available in the next few years.[156]

In hypertension studies lasting up to 2 years, 1,500 mg/day has been used safely without serious adverse effects other than gastrointestinal upset and other effects that quickly resolved.[155] In that study, there was also a decrease in the occurrence of left ventricular hypertrophy. There has been lack of consistency in doses used in studies, although in hypertension it has been used in doses of 750–1,500 mg/day.[155, 160] Stevia has not been studied long-term in diabetes. Because there is lack of regulation, it is best to avoid this product, and the American Dietetic Association does not endorse its use. Women of childbearing age, especially pregnant women, should avoid its use because of the concern of decreased birth weight (from animal data) and mutagenicity.[19]

PINE BARK EXTRACT (*Pinus pinaster*)

Pine bark extract is a unique product that is obtained from French maritime pine bark. It is widely available as Pycnogenol, a standardized extract obtained from pines grown in the Landes de Gascogne forests in southwestern France.[161] The quality of the extract is subject to French regulations and is considered chemically consistent in the available formulations because it is derived from a monoculture that grows for a period of 30–50 years. Since it is grown for such a long time, it is not subject to seasonal variations, and if stored in light-protected containers it is stable for at least 3 years.[161] Pine bark extract has been used for a variety of different disease states and conditions, including varicose veins, coronary artery disease (inhibition of platelet aggregation, hyperlipidemia), and inflammatory conditions such as arthritis, as well as for ergogenic effects and to slow the aging process.[19] In diabetes, it has been used for reduction of blood glucose, retinopathy, and erectile dysfunction.[19] It may be of use in protection against oxidative stress.[161]

Chemical Constituents and Mechanism of Action

The main constituents include procyanidins and phenolic acids.[161] Catechin and epicatechin subunits comprise the procyanidin biopolymers. Pycnogenol specifically contains the monomeric catechin and taxifolin, as well as oligomeric procyanidins. The phenolic components are derived from benzoic and cinnamic acids and include gallic and ferulic as well as other acids.[19, 161]

Pine bark is thought to work as an antioxidant that potently scavenges free radicals and may have a role in regeneration of vitamins E and C. It has anti-inflammatory and immunomodulatory activity and may reduce circulating leukotriene levels. It increases the activity of endothelial nitric oxide synthase and thus may dilate small blood vessels. It has slight inhibition of angiotensin-converting enzyme and some spasmolytic activity. It protects against ultraviolet radiation–induced oxidative stress.[19, 161]

Adverse Effects and Drug Interactions

Most adverse effects are benign and transient. These include gastrointestinal upset, dizziness, and headache.[19, 161] Blood chemistries have shown no changes in liver or renal function.[162] Researchers have noted no changes in vital signs, blood pressure, or electrocardiogram measurements.[163] Thus far, no drug interactions have been reported, but in theory, since it may have immunostimulant effects, it may antagonize the effects of immunosuppressants such as corticosteroids, cyclosporine, or tacrolimus.[19] The same line of reasoning would also apply in suggesting avoidance by people who have autoimmune diseases such as lupus or multiple sclerosis.

Clinical Studies

Although pine bark has been studied for a variety of uses, those most applicable to patients with diabetes are the effects on retinopathy and blood glucose. Five major studies have evaluated its use for retinopathy in a total of 1,289 patients,[164] but only one has been published in English.[162] In this randomized, double-blind study, 20 patients with diabetes were assigned to placebo or 50 mg three times daily of Pycnogenol for 2 months. This was followed by an open-label phase in which another 20 people were treated with the same dose of Pycnogenol for 2 months. Five different ophthalmic assessments were evaluated, including visual acuity, ophthalmoscopy, visual field, fluorangiography, and electroretinogram. For visual acuity determined through a Snellen test, values improved nonsignificantly in the right eye (from 7.57 at baseline to 8.0, $P > 0.05$) and significantly in the left eye (8.1 to 8.67, $P < 0.01$). Ophthalmoscopy was evaluated through an ocular fundus exam, scoring retinal damage on a four-point scale where 0 was normal and 3 showed severe macular hemorrhage. The exam showed improvement in both the right and left eyes. These mean scores declined from 1.6 at baseline to 1.33 at the end in the right eye ($P < 0.01$) and 1.57 to 1.43 in the left eye ($P < 0.05$). Visual field scores were reported as isopters and remained unchanged in both the placebo and Pycnogenol groups. Fluorangiography scores were based on a four-point scale where 0 was normal and 3 was severe. Scores declined significantly in the Pycnogenol group, from 1.7 to 1.3 in the right eye ($P < 0.01$) and from 1.63 to 1.37 in the left eye ($P < 0.01$). Electroretinogram scores measured wave amplitude in the pattern electroretinogram to assess retinal alterations. Scores declined from 1.17 to 0.73 in the right eye ($P < 0.01$) and from 1.03 to 0.57 in the left eye ($P < 0.01$). The researchers provided a subjective judgment that 53% of the Pycnogenol group had "good to very good" efficacy and 47% had "moderate" efficacy.

Two studies have evaluated the use of Pycnogenol for diabetes. The first was a dose-finding open-label trial in 30 patients with type 2 diabetes.[163] After a month-long lifestyle intervention that included diet and exercise, subjects were given successive incremental doses of 50, 100, 200, and 300 mg in 3-week intervals. Every 3 weeks, fasting glucose, 2-hour breakfast postprandial glucose, and A1C were measured. Fasting glucose decreased from 156 mg/dl (8.6 mmol/l) to 136 mg/dl (7.5 mmol/l; $P <$ 0.05) with 200 mg, but the 300-mg dose did not produce any additional decrease. Postprandial glucose decreased from 224 mg/dl (12.5 mmol/l) to 181 mg/dl (10.1 mmol/l), with maximum lowering produced by the 200-mg dose. Once again the 300-mg dose did not produce any additional benefit. Doses up to 300 mg resulted in a continuous A1C decrease from 8% to 7.37%, and the authors reported that significance was achieved after 9–12 weeks with the 200- or 300-mg dose ($P < 0.05$).

The same group of researchers conducted a double-blind, placebo-controlled, randomized, multicenter study in 77 patients with type 2 diabetes.[165] Of the 77 patients, 43 were randomized to placebo and 34 took 100 mg/day Pycnogenol in addition to conventional diabetes medications for 12 weeks. The Pycnogenol group had lower plasma glucose and A1C. Results were reported for median but not mean values. After 12 weeks, the median plasma glucose level decline was 36 mg/dl (2.0 mmol/l) from a baseline of 218.5 mg/dl (12.1 mmol/l; $P < 0.01$). The researchers stated that A1C declined continuously, with a greater decline in the Pycnogenol group, but reported a significant decline only after 1 month of treatment with Pycnogenol. The authors did not report actual A1C values, but stated that the median decline was 0.32% after 1 month ($P < 0.01$) and 0.69% after 3 months (P value not significant).

Summary

Bark derived from maritime pine is primarily available as the extract form in Pycnogenol. This agent has mostly been used for vascular insufficiency, inflammatory disorders, and retinopathy. In smokers, it has also been shown to decrease platelet aggregation.[161] It has a variety of actions that relate to antioxidant effects and dilation of the microcirculation. Adverse effects are mostly benign and include gastric upset and dizziness. It should be avoided in autoimmune diseases such as lupus and multiple sclerosis. Emerging information indicates that Pycnogenol may decrease fasting and postprandial glucose, as well as A1C. There is now some preliminary evidence for use in people with type 2 diabetes. It has been studied short-term for a maximum of 12 weeks in diabetes, and long-term studies are not available. There are problems with study design and reporting results. A potential benefit in diabetes is improvement in retinopathy. The daily dose used for diabetes[163, 165] has been 100–200 mg Pycnogenol. Although there is promising evidence supporting the use of Pycnogenol, there is not enough information to recommend that patients with diabetes use this product.

TEA (*Camellia sinensis*)

A member of the Theaceae family, the tea plant is an evergreen shrub or tree that may grow several feet tall but is usually pruned to 2–5 feet (below 2 meters) when cultivated. The leaves are dark green with serrated edges, and the tree bears white fragrant blossoms.[166] Three types of tea—oolong, black, and green—are produced from the leaves of the tea plant, depending on the processing technique.[167, 168] Oolong tea is partially fermented, black tea is completely fermented, and green tea is not fermented. Oolong and green tea leaves have been used medicinally for a variety of conditions, including diabetes, and are closely related.[19, 168]

Tea, the beverage produced by steeping tea leaves, has been popularly consumed for thousands of years. Medicinally, tea has been used to prevent or treat cardiovascular disease, atherosclerosis, cancer, and obesity; to promote mental alertness, solar radiation protection, dental health; and to provide anti-aging effects.[19, 166, 168, 169] Green tea has been used for hyperlipidemia and hypertension.[19] Oolong tea has also been used for diabetes.[167] Recent evidence indicates that regular consumption of ≥6 cups/day of green tea may lower the risk of developing diabetes.[170]

Chemical Constituents and Mechanism of Action

Tea contains caffeine and polyphenols.[166, 167, 171] The major active components are the polyphenols and are collectively known as catechins.[19, 166, 167] The most significant polyphenols are epigallocatechin gallate, epicatechin gallate, tannins, epigallocatechin, epicatechin, and gallocatechin gallate.[19, 166, 171]

The polyphenols have varying properties including antioxidant, anti-inflammatory, and anticancer effects.[19, 168] Antioxidant effects are related to the chemical structure of aromatic rings and hydroxyl groups. The hydroxyl groups bind and neutralize free radical groups. Antioxidant effects have been thought to diminish oxidative damage and lipid peroxidation in smokers.[168] The catechins also inhibit prostaglandin and leukotriene production.[166] Cardiovascular protection may be a result of decreased LDL oxidation by some of the components in tea.[168] Some of the components may also increase metabolic rate and fat oxidation and may have some anti-obesity effects. Adiponectin levels are decreased in individuals with cardiovascular disease, obesity, and diabetes, and oolong tea has been shown to increase adiponectin levels.[172] Another ingredient in green tea, theanine, has been thought to provide some immunoprotection against infectious agents, as well as some slight blood pressure reduction, chemotherapy modulation, relaxation, and neuroprotection.[173]

The caffeine content has varying effects, including increased resting energy expenditure and cellular thermogenesis, increased or decreased blood glucose, and varying effects on blood pressure.[19] Specific polyphenols, particularly those found in tea, are thought to enhance insulin activity, which may be responsible for some of the benefits in diabetes.[171]

Adverse Effects and Drug Interactions

The main adverse effects include caffeine toxicity, which manifests as insomnia, anxiety, restlessness, nausea, and tachycardia.[19] Use by pregnant women should be minimal because of unknown fetal effects. Lactating women should also limit tea consumption because of problems with irritability or sleep disturbances in the infant.[166] Overdose may result in catecholamine release and thus cause anxiety.[19] In weight-loss supplements (not in beverage form), there are several cases of hepatotoxicity from products containing green tea.[174]

Oolong and green tea may decrease absorption of iron from foods.[19] The aluminum content in green tea may adversely affect people with renal dysfunction, since aluminum accumulation may eventually result in neurotoxicity.[168] Adding milk (including soy milk) or creamers to tea decreases the insulin potentiation, although adding lemon has no effect.[171] There are potential interactions between tea and different lab tests or procedures. For instance, tea may interfere with dipyridamole thallium tests because of the caffeine content. False elevations in uric acid have been reported as well as increased vanillylmandelic acid concentrations.[19] Disease interactions may include worsening anxiety or worsening glaucoma due to increased intraocular pressure.[19]

There are many potential drug interactions with either green or oolong tea. The caffeine content may result in toxicity when tea is combined with sympathomimetics or amphetamines, or with CAM supplements that cause stimulant effects, such as ephedra and bitter orange. Other agents that may increase caffeine effects are ethanol, cimetidine, disulfiram, oral contraceptives, estrogens, certain quinolones, terbinafine, theophylline, verapamil, fluconazole, and fluvoxamine. In combination with monoamine oxidase (MAO) inhibitors, increased blood pressure and heart rate may occur. The caffeine content may decrease serum concentrations of clozapine and lithium. Caffeine may increase bleeding risk when used with antiplatelet drugs or CAM supplements that have antiplatelet effects.[19] Although tea has been reported to have antiplatelet effects, green tea may antagonize the antiplatelet effects of warfarin because of its vitamin K content.[19, 124] Nicotine may result in additive central nervous system effects when combined with tea, and the calming effect of certain drugs, such as pentobarbital, may be negated by tea consumption. There is a theoretical additive hypoglycemic effect if combined with insulin or secretagogues.

Clinical Studies

Tea has been widely studied. In one trial evaluating oolong tea in type 2 diabetes, 20 individuals on diabetes agents were assigned in a randomized crossover fashion to drink 1,500 ml (~6.25 cups) of oolong tea or water daily (consumed five times per day) for 1 month.[167] Following a 2-week washout from tea consumption, patients were randomized to tea or water for 1 month, followed by another 2-week washout and then crossover to the other group for 30 days. Plasma glucose was measured after each washout and treatment period. Mean plasma glucose decreased from 229 mg/dl (12.7 mmol/l) at baseline to 162 mg/dl (9.0 mmol/l; $P < 0.001$) in the tea group. Fructosamine also decreased from 410 μmol/l at baseline to 323 μmol/l after treatment ($P < 0.01$).

In another randomized crossover trial, oolong tea was administered to 22 patients with type 2 diabetes.[172] Twelve patients had a history of myocardial infarction, and 10 had angina. After a 2-week washout, patients were randomized to 4 weeks of water or 1,000 ml/day (4.5 cups) of oolong tea for 4 weeks. Patients then also had another 2-week washout and were crossed over to the other group for 4 weeks. A1C levels decreased from a baseline of 7.23% to 6.99% ($P < 0.05$), and glucose decreased from 173 mg/dl (9.6 mmol/l) to 156 mg/dl (8.7 mmol/l). However, the difference was not significant. LDL cholesterol decreased slightly (123 mg/dl [3.2 mmol/l] to 117 mg/dl [3.0 mmol/l]), although the results were not significant. Total cholesterol also decreased (209 mg/dl [5.4 mmol/l] to 197 mg/dl [5.1 mmol/l], $P < 0.01$). Adiponectin increased significantly (6.26 μg/ml to 6.88 μg/ml, $P < 0.05$). Another study showed that when 240 subjects with hyperlipidemia were given a green tea extract for 12 weeks, total and LDL cholesterol decreased significantly (11.3% and 16.4%, respectively; $P = 0.01$ for both).[175]

Summary

Next to water, tea is the most highly consumed beverage in the world. Some types used in diabetes include oolong and green tea. They differ in caffeine and polyphenol content, although green and oolong tea are closely related. There are many reasons patients may drink tea for health-related purposes, including antioxidant, anticancer, and anti-aging effects. People with diabetes may drink tea to decrease glucose and lipids and to lose weight. Numerous drug, herb, lab, and disease interactions are possible. As a beverage, tea may not be problematic unless consumed in excessive quantities, and then caffeine's adverse effects may predominate. Including green tea as an ingredient in supplements for weight loss may result in hepatotoxicity.[174] For diabetes the results are preliminary, although it is intriguing that a recent 5-year observational study found that consumption of ≥ 6 cups/day of green tea was associated with a decreased risk of type 2 diabetes.[170] However, in this study, there was no positive benefit of oolong tea. Although oolong tea has been reported to decrease plasma glucose and fructosamine, only short-term study information is available. If a patient wishes to consume oolong or green tea, the daily consumption should be about 6 cups a day. Pregnant and lactating women should limit consumption. Overall, supplements containing tea should be avoided.

BILBERRY (*Vaccinium myrtillus*)

Bilberry is a plant that originated in North and Central Europe.[75] It is related to the American blueberry, cranberry, and huckleberry and is used to prepare jellies, pies, and cobblers. In medieval times, it was thought to be useful for inducing menstruation. Other uses have included treatment of kidney stones and typhoid fever.[75] Two forms of bilberry are used: the dried fruit and the leaf.[62] The dried fruit is used to treat diarrhea,[62] to improve visual acuity and night vision, and to prevent cataracts[176] and varicose veins.[19] The dried fruit extract has been used to treat diabetes, arthritis, and circulatory disorders.[19, 62, 75] In folk medicine, bilberry is used as a blood glucose–reducing drug and is therefore a common constituent in antidiabetic teas.[140]

Chemical Constituents and Mechanism of Action

Catechin tannins in the fruit are thought to have astringent effects.[62] Anthocyanosides are bioflavonoids, the chemical constituents in bilberry fruit that are thought to decrease vascular permeability and redistribute microvascular blood flow.[75] These substances are similar to some of the agents found in grape seed and are proposed as the active components in vision- and vascular-related claims. Other active ingredients include flavonoids such as quercitrin and isoquercitrin, as well as phenolic acids.[140] Animal research indicates that the mechanism of action of bilberry in diabetes may be related to the high chromium content in the bilberry leaf (9 ppm).[140] The leaf also contains another substance, neomirtilline, that may decrease blood glucose.[177] Research is needed to determine whether this proposed mechanism of action in diabetes is valid.

Adverse Effects and Drug Interactions

Most of the reported adverse effects of bilberry have been benign, such as mild digestive distress, skin rashes, and drowsiness. There are no known drug interactions, but it does inhibit platelet aggregation and thus may interact with drugs or CAM supplements that also possess antiplatelet activity. Since it may affect blood glucose, a theoretical additive hypoglycemic effect may occur with secretagogues. If an alcoholic extract is used, a disulfiram reaction may occur.[124] In animals, high doses have resulted in initial cachexia and excitation, followed by eventual death with prolonged use.[62]

Clinical Studies

In spite of early enthusiasm and speculation during World War II about the beneficial effect of bilberry preserves in improving night vision in Royal Air Force pilots, this effect has not been demonstrated in controlled trials. One randomized, double-blind, placebo-controlled study was done in 15 men recruited from a naval air station.[178] The subjects were given 160 mg bilberry extract containing 25% anthocyanosides or placebo three times a day for 21 days. There were no differences between the groups in night visual acuity or night contrast sensitivity. In another randomized, double-blind, placebo-controlled trial, 16 men with normal vision were given three different doses of anthocyanosides once daily (12, 24, or 36 mg) or placebo, with a 2-week washout between doses.[179] There were no differences in night vision between the anthocyanoside groups and placebo. Another randomized, double-blind, placebo-controlled study evaluated three different night-vision tests in 18 healthy male volunteers.[180] The subjects received 12 or 24 mg anthocyanosides or placebo twice daily for 4 days, with a 2-week washout between doses. Once again there was no difference between the treatment and placebo groups.

In a trial in streptozotocin-induced diabetic rats, 4 days of bilberry leaf administration resulted in consistent decreases in plasma glucose by 26%.[177] In a double-blind, placebo-controlled, trial published in Italian, bilberry extract (160 mg twice daily; 115 mg anthocyanosides daily) was administered to 14 patients with retinopathy related to diabetes and/or hypertension.[181] The 11 patients on bilberry and 12 patients on placebo were treated for 1 month. The bilberry group showed significant improvement in ophthalmoscopic parameters.

Summary

Although bilberry is widely used, it is important that clinicians and patients know there is not much published evidence for its use in diabetes or for visual improvement. The benefit in diabetes may be related to chromium content in the leaf. It is a relatively benign agent, although in animals, toxicity with high doses or prolonged use has been reported. Standard doses of the dried ripe berries are 20–60 g daily. Decoctions are prepared by placing mashed berries in cold water and simmering for several minutes. The liquid is then strained and consumed.[19] The leaf is prepared as a tea. Bilberry extract, 160 mg twice daily, has been useful in retinopathy.[181] Animal data has shown benefit in lowering blood glucose and triglycerides,[177] but there are no trials in humans to document efficacy in diabetes.[19] Preliminary evidence has shown that bilberry may help prevent cataracts,[177] which may be of importance to diabetes patients because they are more prone to cataracts. Other preliminary evidence indicates bilberry use may be of benefit in retinopathy.[181] Although there are European studies of bilberry for retinopathy, they are not published in English. Even though it may be a benign agent, there is insufficient evidence to promote bilberry use.

MILK THISTLE (*Silybum marianum*)

Milk thistle is a member of the aster family (Asteraceae or Compositae), which also includes daisies and thistles.[182] Milk thistle grows well in North America and reaches 5–10 feet (about 2–3 meters) in height, with large prickly leaves that secrete a milk sap when broken.[183] It bears pink flowers that are ridged with sharp spines. Medicinal constituents are found in the fruit, seeds, and leaves of the plant.

Milk thistle has been used for thousands of years and is noted in ancient Greek and Roman references.[75] It has been used extensively for various hepatic disorders, such as hepatotoxicity secondary to acute and chronic viral hepatitis or alcoholic cirrhosis. Other uses have been to treat *Amanita phalloides* poisoning and to attenuate hepatotoxic effects of certain medications.[182] It is used for uterine complaints and stimulation of menstrual flow. In Europe it is also consumed as a vegetable.[19] Its use has been proposed in diabetes to diminish insulin resistance.[184]

Chemical Constituents and Mechanism of Action

Milk thistle contains silymarin, which is composed of three main constituents: silybin, silychristine, and silidianin. Silybin is thought to have the most potent biological activity.[183] Silymarin is extracted with 95% ethyl alcohol, which yields a bright yellow fluid.[183]

There are several proposed mechanisms of action of milk thistle in hepatic disease.[182] One mechanism is inhibition of hepatotoxin binding to hepatocyte membrane receptor sites, resulting in hepatocyte stabilization. Another mechanism is decreased glutathione oxidation, which may replenish diminished glutathione levels in the liver and intestines. It also has antioxidant activity to protect against toxic free radicals and may enhance protein synthesis and result in hepatocyte regeneration.[182] Other possible effects are regulation of inflammatory mediators such as tumor necrosis factor, nitrous oxide, and inflammatory interleukins.[185] It may also increase lymphocyte proliferation and inhibit leukotriene formation.[185] Thus, milk thistle is often known as a cytoprotectant. It may be of benefit in insulin resistance associated with hepatic damage. One theory is that lipoperoxidation may adversely affect patients with diabetes and therefore replenishment of malondialdehyde (MDA) concentrations may improve diabetes.[184]

Adverse Effects and Drug Interactions

Side effects of milk thistle include dose-related diarrhea because of increased bile flow.[186] A few case reports have been reported by the Australian Adverse Drug Reactions Advisory Committee that include intermittent episodes of severe sweating, gastrointestinal upset, and weakness that recurred on rechallenge.[187] Other adverse effects include possible allergic reactions in people who are sensitive to ragweed, chrysanthemums, marigolds, and daisies.[19, 182]

No known adverse interactions have been reported with milk thistle. However, it may somewhat attenuate phase I and phase II hepatic metabolism[75] and may slightly inhibit CYP 3A4, 2D6, and 2E1.[185] Beneficial interactions, however, have included attenuation of hepatotoxic effects of acetaminophen, antipsychotics, halothane, and alcohol.[19, 182]

Clinical Studies

The studies evaluating milk thistle have had serious design problems. Many studies are open-label, involve small patient numbers, lack control groups, use different doses, lack well-defined end points, or involve varying hepatic disease severity. Several studies have evaluated effects of milk thistle on hepatic disease with inconclusive results.[183] A recent evaluation of randomized clinical trials of patients with alcoholic liver disease or hepatitis indicated that in high-quality clinical trials, milk thistle does not positively impact hepatic-related mortality.[188] Also, milk thistle did not significantly influence the clinical course of patients with hepatitis or alcoholic disease.

Milk thistle was evaluated in a randomized, open-label trial in 60 patients with type 2 diabetes and cirrhosis.[184] Two groups of patients on insulin were compared. One group of 30 received 600 mg/day silymarin, and 30 patients received placebo for 12 months. Some studied end points included fasting blood glucose, mean daily blood glucose, A1C, insulin dose, fasting insulin, and MDA levels (since this is a peroxidation marker that is elevated in cirrhosis). Results were significant in the silymarin group but not in the control group. Mean fasting glucose declined from 190 mg/dl (10.6 mmol/l) at baseline to 165 mg/dl (9.2 mmol/l) at 12 months ($P < 0.01$ vs. baseline). Mean daily glucose decreased from 202 mg/dl (11.2 mmol/l) at baseline to 172 mg/dl (9.6 mmol/l) at end point ($P < 0.01$ vs. baseline). A1C decreased from 7.9% at baseline to 7.2% at end point ($P < 0.01$ vs. baseline). Mean daily insulin requirement decreased significantly from 55 units a day to 42 units a day at end point ($P < 0.01$ vs. baseline). Mean fasting insulin levels declined significantly in the silymarin-treated patients ($P < 0.01$ vs. baseline). Mean MDA level decreased from 2.2 μmol/ml to 1.55 μmol/ml at 12 months ($P < 0.01$). This was close to the upper limits of normal levels found in patients with healthy livers (1.5 μmol/ml). In the control group, there was a slight nonsignificant increase in MDA.

In another 4-month, double-blind study, 25 people were randomized to 300 mg twice daily of silymarin seed extract, and 26 were randomized to placebo.[189] Silymarin was added to a regimen of metformin and glibenclamide. Fasting blood glucose declined significantly from 156 mg/dl (8.7 mmol/l) to 133 mg/dl (7.4 mmol/l) in the silymarin group ($P < 0.001$) after 4 months and increased significantly in the placebo group

(167 mg/dl [9.3 mmol/l] at baseline to 188 mg/dl [10.4 mmol/l], $P <$ 0.0001). The silymarin group had a decrease in A1C from 7.8% to 6.8% after 4 months ($P < 0.001$), and the placebo had an increase in A1C from 8.3% to 9.5% ($P < 0.0001$). LDL cholesterol and triglycerides also decreased significantly in the silymarin group (140 mg/dl [3.6 mmol/l] to 123 mg/dl [3.2 mmol/l], $P = 0.005$; and 284 mg/dl [3.2 mmol/l] to 211 mg/dl [2.4 mmol/l], $P = 0.004$, respectively).

Summary

Although milk thistle is an extensively studied agent, problems with study design make it impossible to routinely recommend this agent. However, even long-term use has attested to the safety of milk thistle. It is an agent that has also been used for nonalcoholic steatohepatitis.[190] Adverse events are rare, although gastrointestinal effects and cross-allergic reactions may occur with members of the daisy and ragweed family. Milk thistle may diminish toxic effects of hepatotoxic drugs. The typical dose of milk thistle for liver disease is 200 mg three times daily. Milk thistle extract should be standardized to contain 70% silymarin (140 mg silymarin). Since phosphatidylcholine enhances oral absorption, preparations containing this ingredient may be dosed at 100 mg/day.[182] Parenteral doses have been used in Europe. Doses differ from those used in clinical studies, which ranged from 280 mg/day to 800 mg/day. Although there is some potential benefit for use in diabetes as a hepatoprotectant or for nonalcoholic steatohepatitis, there are only small studies in patients with type 2 diabetes; therefore, routine use is not recommended.

Table 1. Botanical CAM Supplements Used to Treat Diabetes

Botanical Product	Chemical Constituents	Mechanism of Action	Side Effects & Drug Interactions
Cinnamon	Hydroxychalcone [64]	• ↑ insulin sensitivity • ↑ cell/tissue glucose uptake • Promotes glycogen synthesis [64]	*Side effects:* • No side effects reported; may cause irritation or dermatitis if used topically [62] *Drug interactions:* • May ↓ blood glucose if used with secretagogues [19]

Gymnema	• Gymnemosides
	• Saponins
	• Stigmasterol
	• Amino acid derivatives
	  - betaine
	  - choline
	  - trimethylamine
	[70]
		• Impairs ability to discriminate "sweet" taste
		• ↑ enzymes promoting glucose uptake
		• May stimulate β-cells
		• May ↑ β-cell number
		• May ↑ insulin release
		[19,71–73,75]
			Side effects:
			• None reported
			• May cause hypoglycemia [19,75]
			Drug interactions:
			• Possible hypoglycemia if combined with secretagogues [19,75]

(Continued)

Table 1. (*Continued*)

Botanical Product	Chemical Constituents	Mechanism of Action	Side Effects & Drug Interactions

Fenugreek	• Saponins
	• Glycosides
	• Seeds contain
	  - alkaloids
	  - 4-hydroxyisoleucine
	  - fenugreekine
	[19,75,77–79]
		• Delayed gastric emptying
		• Slowed carbohydrate absorption
		• Glucose transport inhibition
		• ↑ insulin receptors
		• Improved peripheral glucose utilization
		• Possible stimulation of insulin secretion
		[19,77–79]
			Side effects:
			• Diarrhea, gas
			• Uterine contractions
			• Allergic reactions
			[19,76]
			Drug interactions:
			• May ↑ anticoagulant effects of warfarin or herbs with anticoagulant activity (boldo, garlic, ginger) [19,80]

Bitter Melon	• Momordin • Charantin • Polypeptide P • Vicine [19,75,85]	• Hypoglycemic action • Tissue glucose uptake; glycogen synthesis • Inhibition of enzymes involved in glucose production • Enhanced glucose oxidation of glucose-6-phosphate-dehydrogenase (G6PDH) pathway [19,85]	*Side effects:* • Gastrointestinal discomfort • Hypoglycemic coma • Favism • Hemolytic anemia in persons with G6PDH deficiency • Contains known abortifacients (α- and β-momorcharin) • Seeds have produced vomiting, death in children [19,85]

Ginseng	Ginsenosides [19,94]	• May ↓ carbohydrate absorption in portal circulation • May ↑ glucose transport and uptake • Modulation of insulin secretion [19,75,91,94–98]	*Drug interactions:* • Hypoglycemia when used with sulfonylureas [87] *Side effects:* • Insomnia, headache, restlessness • ↑ blood pressure or heart rate • Mastalgia • Mood changes, nervousness [19,75,91,94] *Drug interactions:* • ↓ warfarin effectiveness • ↓ diuretic effectiveness • Additive estrogenic effects • Possible ↑ effects of certain analgesics and antidepressants • Possible additive hypoglycemia with secretagogues [19,75,94]
Nopal	•Mucopolysaccharide fibers • Pectin [19,75]	• Slows carbohydrate absorption • ↓ lipid absorption • Possibly ↑ insulin sensitivity [19,75,107]	*Side effects:* • Diarrhea, nausea, abdominal fullness • ↑ stool volume [19,75,105]

(Continued)

Table 1. (*Continued*)

Botanical Product	Chemical Constituents	Mechanism of Action	Side Effects & Drug Interactions
			Drug interactions: • Improved blood glucose and insulin with sulfonylureas (without hypoglycemia) [19,75,106]
Aloe	• Aloe gel contains glucomannan (polysaccharide similar to guar gum and glycoprotein) [19,109]	• Fiber may promote glucose uptake [19,109]	*Side effects:* • None reported *Drug interactions:* • Possible hypoglycemia if combined with secretagogues [19] • Intraoperative blood loss in surgery patients where sevoflurance was used [111]
Banaba	Corsolic acid and ellagitannin called lagerstroemin [113–115]	• Ellagitannins bind to protein kinase A subunit • May stimulate glucose uptake and have insulin-like activity (secondary to activation of insulin receptor tyrosine kinase or inhibition of tyrosine phosphatase) [113–115]	*Side effects:* • None reported *Drug interactions:* • Possible hypoglycemia if combined with secretagogues [19]

Caiapo	Acidic glycoprotein [116–118]	• Improved insulin sensitivity • ↓ insulin resistance [116–118]	*Side effects:* • Constipation, gastrointestinal pain, meteorism [116] *Drug interactions:* • Possible hypoglycemia if combined with secretagogues [19]
Ivy Gourd	• Unknown active ingredients; trace alkaloids • Contains beta-carotene [120–122]	• Suppresses glucose-6-phosphatase (enzyme involved in glucose production) • Insulin-like activity [121,122]	*Side effects:* • Theoretical allergic reaction to plant component [19] *Drug interactions:* • None reported • Possible hypoglycemia if combined with secretagogues [19]
Holy Basil	• Eugenol • Linalool • Methyl chavicol (estragole) • Other ingredients - caryophyllene - monoterpenes, sesquiterpenes, phenylpropanes [124,127]	• May improve pancreatic β-cell function and enhance insulin secretion [124,127]	*Side effects:* • None reported in humans; may decrease sperm count per animal data [128,129] • Possible bleeding reactions, per animal data [130]

(*Continued*)

Table 1. (*Continued*)

Botanical Product	Chemical Constituents	Mechanism of Action	Side Effects & Drug Interactions
			Drug interactions: • None reported; possible hypoglycemia if combined with secretagogues • Theoretical additive sedation with sedatives related to barbiturates • Possible bleeding if combined with antiplatelets such as aspirin, warfarin, or CAM supplements with antiplatelet effects [19,130]

Vijayasar	• (-)Epicatechin
	• Phenolic components
	  - marsupin
	  - ptorosupin
	  - pterostilbene
	[131,134]
		• ↑ islet cyclic adenosine monophosphate, which may ↑ insulin release
		• Facilitate conversion of proinsulin to insulin
		• Insulin-like effects
		[131,134]
			Side effects:
			• None reported
			[134]
			Drug interactions:
			• None reported; theoretical additive hypoglycemia with secretagogues
			[19,134]

Jambolan	• Gallic acid • Ellagic acid • Corilagin • Quercetin • Tannins [124]	• Seeds may have hypoglycemic effects • Seeds may also have antihypertensive and anti-inflammatory actions [124]	*Side effects:* • None reported • In animals may see ↓ activity and other CNS effects [124,137] *Drug interactions:* • None reported; theoretical additive hypoglycemia with secretagogues • Theoretical additive effects with CNS depressants [124]
Blonde Psyllium	• Mix of acidic/neutral polysaccharides with galacturonic acid [139]	• Formation of viscous gel that slows intestinal absorption of glucose • Delayed gastric emptying • Carbohydrate sequestering • May also lower dietary fat absorption [141,142]	*Side effects:* • Allergies • Swallowing disorders [19,140] *Drug interactions:* • Binding reactions, thus ↓ absorption of other drugs (carbamazepine, iron supplements, riboflavin) • Possible additive hypoglycemia with secretagogues [19]

(*Continued*)

Table 1. (*Continued*)

Botanical Product	Chemical Constituents	Mechanism of Action	Side Effects & Drug Interactions

Glucomannan	• Polysaccharide consisting of
	  - glucose
	  - mannose
	
	[75]
		• May delay glucose and cholesterol absorption
		• May ↓ hepatic cholesterol synthesis
		
		[148]
			Side effects:
			• Esophageal obstruction reported with tablets (not powders or capsules) [19,124]
			
			Drug interactions:
			• May bind oil-soluble vitamins (A, D, E, K)
			• Possible additive hypoglycemia with secretagogues
			• Possible additive lipid lowering with antihyperlipidemics [19,124]

Guar Gum	• Polysaccharide consisting of - galactomannan [75]	• Hypoglycemic activity due to altered GI transit and delayed glucose absorption • Lipid-lowering activity due to ↓ lipid absorption and ↑ bile excretion [75]	*Side effects:* • GI upset • Esophageal obstruction [19] *Drug interactions:* • Possible additive hypoglycemia with secretagogues [19] • Possible additive lipid lowering with antihyperlipidemics [150] • May ↓ absorption of drugs taken at the same time [19]

| Stevia | • Diterpene glycosides, including
  - stevioside
  - sulcoside
  - rebaudiosides
• Steviolbioside [124,157] | • ↑ glucose utilization through inhibition of oxidative phosphorylation
• ↑ glucose utilization
• May inhibit gluconeogenesis
• Possible ↑ insulin secretion [157,158]
• May also block calcium channels [155]
• Vasodilation, diuretic activity [19] | *Side effects:*
• GI upset
• Headache
• Asthenia
• Myalgia [155]
• Possible allergic reactions in persons allergic to Asteraceae or Compositae family (ragweed, daisies, etc.) [19]
• In animals, mutagenicity and nephrotoxicity [124]
Drug interactions:
• Possible additive hypoglycemia if combined with secretagogues [19]
• Possible additive hypotension with calcium channel blockers [155] |

(Continued)

Table 1. (*Continued*)

Botanical Product	Chemical Constituents	Mechanism of Action	Side Effects & Drug Interactions
Pine Bark Extract	• Procyanidins - catechin - epicatechin • Phenolic acids - gallic acid - ferulic acid [161]	• Antioxidant effect - Free radical scavenging • Anti-inflammatory and immunomodulatory effects [19,161]	*Side effects:* • GI upset • Headache [19,161] *Drug interactions:* • May antagonize effects of immunosuppresants (steroids, cyclosporine, etc.) [19]
Tea	• Polyphenols (catechins) - epigallocatechin gallate - epicatechin gallate - epigallocatechin - epicatechin - gallocatechin gallate - tannins • Caffeine [166,167,171]	• Antioxidant effects • Anti-inflammatory effects • Some polyphenols may enhance insulin activity [19,168,171,173]	*Side effects:* • Caffeine toxicity (insomnia, anxiety, restlessness) [19] • Hepatotoxicity from green tea products [174] • ↑ aluminum absorption and subsequent neurotoxicity [168] • False ↑ in uric acid [19] • Interference with dipyridamole thallium tests [19] • Glaucoma worsening [19] • Possible additive hypoglycemia if combined with secretagogues [19]

Drug interactions:
- Increased activation if combined with stimulants [19]
- ↓ absorption of iron in foods [19]
- ↑ caffeine effects if combined with many drugs such as cimetidine, disulfiram, oral estrogens, theophylline, fluconazole, and many others [19]
- Green tea may antagonize warfarin effects [19,124]

Bilberry
- Anthocyanosides (bioflavonoids)
- Chromium in bilberry leaf
- Neomirtilline

[19,62,75,140,177]

- May ↓ vascular permeability and redistribute microvascular blood flow [19,75]
- Per animal research, chromium content in leaf may contribute to hypoglycemic activity [140]

Side effects:
- Mild gastrointestinal distress
- Skin rashes [19,75]

Drug interactions:
- None known but possible additive hypoglycemia with secretagogues [124]
- Possible disulfiram reactions if an alcoholic extract is used [124]

(Continued)

Table 1. (*Continued*)

Botanical Product	Chemical Constituents	Mechanism of Action	Side Effects & Drug Interactions
Milk thistle	• Silymarin, containing silybin, silychristine, and silidianin [182,183]	• Inhibition of hepatotoxin binding to hepatocyte membrane receptors • ↓ glutathione oxidation (may then replenish diminished glutathione levels in liver and intestines) [182,183] • Regulation of inflammatory mediators (tumor necrosis factor, inflammatory interleukins) [185] • May ↑ lymphocyte proliferation and ↓ leukotriene formation [185]	*Side effects:* • Diarrhea, weakness, sweating [19,186,187] • Possible allergic reactions if also allergic to ragweed, marigolds, daisies, chrysanthemums [19,182] *Drug interactions:* • No adverse interactions known • Beneficial interactions with hepatotoxic agents such as acetaminophen, antipsychotics, alcohol [182]

3.

Nonbotanical CAM Supplements to Treat Diabetes

It is important for clinicians to have an appreciation of the many diverse forms of supplements that patients have used for diabetes. Along with supplements of botanical origin, many nonbotanical products are available and have been used either alone or in combination with conventional medications. Table 2 (on page 107) provides a brief summary of the information in this section.

CHROMIUM

Chromium is a trace element found in trivalent or hexavalent forms. The hexavalent form is a carcinogen with toxicity occurring only in industrial exposure and is not found in natural foods. Trivalent forms include chromium picolinate, nicotinate, and chloride. The trivalent form is nontoxic and is found in certain foods such as high-bran cereals, whole grains, broccoli and other fresh vegetables, egg yolks, brewer's yeast, meat, nuts, cheese, and certain wines and beers.[191] Many years ago, brewer's yeast was thought to contain an unrecognized dietary ingredient known as glucose tolerance factor, or GTF. In animal research, GTF was thought to be an essential nutrient to maintain normal glucose metabolism.[192] Brewer's yeast contains abundant chromium, which was thought to be part of this organic complex. However, the term GTF is no longer used.

Chromium deficiency may occur when a person is on total parenteral nutrition,[193] is pregnant, or has a poor diet, high glucose intake, or poor glucose control.[191, 194] There is currently no evidence to show that chromium deficiency rates are higher in people with diabetes than in the general population,[19, 75] but diabetes has developed in experimental animals with low chromium levels.[191]

Chromium has been used for weight loss, for its ergogenic properties, and for improving lipid and glycemic control.[19, 75] Since increased chromium excretion may occur with steroid use, chromium supplementation has been used to reverse corticosteroid-induced diabetes.[195]

The Food and Nutrition Board of the Institute of Medicine has determined there is not sufficient evidence to set an estimated average requirement for chromium.[196] An adequate intake was set based on estimated mean intakes. The adequate intake is 35 μg/day for young men and 25 μg/day for young women. Because few serious adverse effects are reported from excess intake of chromium in food, no tolerable upper level has been established. Since there is no accurate assay for body chromium stores, it is difficult to determine when an individual has chromium deficiency and how supplementation may affect the deficiency.

Mechanism of Action

The trivalent chromium form is used therapeutically. The exact mechanism by which chromium affects glucose metabolism is unknown. Current knowledge is based on effects of chromium deprivation and supplementation. It is known that chromium is an essential mineral for glucose metabolism. Supplementation is likely beneficial in deficiency states. The trivalent form is believed to play a role in enhancing cellular effects of insulin.[191] Chromium may affect insulin activity through enhanced activity of tyrosine kinase, the enzyme required for phosphorylation. Thus chromium may improve insulin action by enhancing tyrosine kinase activity. In effect, chromium may increase insulin receptor number, insulin binding, and/or insulin activation. The proposed overall effect of chromium may be to increase insulin receptor or β-cell sensitivity.[191, 193]

Adverse Effects and Drug Interactions

Reported side effects of chromium are related to excessive consumption and include renal toxicity, including acute renal failure caused by severe interstitial nephritis; severe systemic illness, including hemolysis; thrombocytopenia; hepatic dysfunction; and renal failure.[197–199] Other adverse effects have included dermatologic reactions[200] and mood disturbances.[19] However, studies have demonstrated the safety of large doses of chromium picolinate[201] and long-term administration.[202]

There are unique effects of other drugs on chromium. Steroids may deplete chromium, and histamine blockers (famotidine) and proton pump inhibitors (omeprazole) may block chromium absorption.[19] Certain drugs and vitamins, such as anti-inflammatory drugs (ibuprofen) and vitamin C, may increase chromium absorption.[19] Coadministration with zinc may decrease absorption of both nutrients. Additive hypoglycemia with insulin or insulin secretagogues is a theoretical possibility.[19]

Clinical Studies

Positive effects of chromium have been shown in patients with type 1 or type 2 diabetes, gestational diabetes, or impaired glucose tolerance.[191] Studies have shown variable benefits for diabetes and hyperlipidemia. Lower toenail chromium concentrations have been found in subjects with increased risk of diabetes.[203] Trials with negative results used less-bioavailable forms of chromium, such as chromium chloride or chromium-rich yeast.

In a randomized, double-blind, placebo-controlled trial in 180 Chinese patients, fasting blood glucose and A1C levels decreased significantly in the group taking 1,000 μg/day of chromium picolinate compared with the 200 μg/day group and placebo group.[201] Patients were randomized to placebo or to 100 μg twice daily or 500 μg twice daily of chromium picolinate for 4 months. Fasting glucose decreased significantly in the 1,000 μg/day group at 2 and 4 months (baseline numbers were not given; results were reported in graph form). The authors reported that at 4 months, fasting glucose was 158 mg/dl (8.8 mmol/l) in the placebo group, 155 mg/dl (8.6 mmol/l) in the 200 μg/day group, and 128 mg/dl (7.1 mmol/l) in the 1,000 μg/day group ($P < 0.05$ for the 1,000-μg group vs. the other two groups). From graph interpretation, baseline A1C was 9.4% in the two chromium groups and 9.2% in the placebo group. After 4 months, A1C was 8.5%, 7.5%, and 6.6%, respectively, in the placebo, 200 μg/day, and 1,000 μg/day groups. Thus, A1C decreased by 2.8% in the highest dose group and by 1.9% in the other chromium group ($P < 0.05$, reduction for both chromium groups vs. placebo). Overall, effects were dose-dependent and were seen at 2 and 4 months.

A recent meta-analysis of randomized controlled trials evaluating the effects of chromium use on insulin and glucose reported that data are inconclusive and more studies are needed to evaluate the role of chromium supplementation in diabetes.[204] Another review evaluated several studies, including those with long-term administration of chromium in higher doses, and found that overall chromium supplementation may be beneficial.[191] Two recent studies have shown negative results. One study used 800 μg/day of chromium picolinate for 3 months in patients with impaired glucose tolerance[205] and the other study used 1,000 μg/day of chromium picolinate in obese, insulin-treated type 2 diabetes.[206] However, critics have stated that the chromium dose used was suboptimal because the chromium picolinate used contained only 12.4% chromium picolinate.[207]

Summary

Chromium is a trace element that is deficient in certain circumstances, possibly including diabetes. Chromium may work as an insulin sensitizer and enhance β-cell function. However, studies of chromium in impaired glucose tolerance, type 1, and type 2 diabetes have shown variable effects. The landmark study done in Chinese patients[201] showed benefit, but this group of patients may have different dietary chromium intake than the average American population. These patients were much leaner than many typical diabetes patients in the U.S. Although higher doses of chromium have been studied and shown to be more effective, a typical dose is 200 μg/day.[19] Short-term, dose-related responses have been shown, and doses up to 1,000 μg/day for 64 months have not shown adverse effects,[202] but more study is needed. Results from chromium research are not conclusive, particularly in light of lack of information regarding the most appropriate biomarkers for chromium or the most appropriate formulation. If used, picolinate salt appears to be the most appropriate form. Supplements containing chromium picolinate in combination with biotin are undergoing extensive study.[208] In August 2005 the FDA authorized a qualified health claim that chromium picolinate may reduce the risk of insulin resistance, based on a small study.[209, 210] The official American Diabetes Association (ADA) stance is that there is no conclusive evidence demonstrating that chromium supplementation in diabetes should be done.[211] However, its popularity continues, and overall side effects have not been serious.

VANADIUM

Vanadium is a trace element found in several spices and foods, including black pepper, parsley, dill seeds, mushrooms, spinach, and shellfish.[212] It is also found in cereals, sunflower seeds, grains, wine, and beer.[213] In 1831, a Swedish chemist named the compound *vanadis*, a nickname for the Norse goddess of beauty, youth, and luster, because the salts have beautiful colors.[19, 212, 213] Vanadium has been used for hyperlipidemia and heart disease and for cancer prevention. Although it has been used for bodybuilding, it has not been found to be effective.[214] It has also been used for diabetes.

Vanadium intake is reported to range from 6 μg/day to 18 μg/day.[196] Appropriate indicators for establishing an adequate intake for vanadium are not currently available. The estimate of tolerable upper level for vanadium for adults is 1.8 mg/day.[196] Vanadium is available as different salts. Vanadyl sulfate contains 31%, sodium metavanadate contains 42%, and sodium orthovanadate contains 28% elemental vanadium.[19]

Mechanism of Action

Vanadium may function in various parts of the insulin signaling pathway.[213, 215] It is also thought to have direct insulin-mimetic activity and may increase tissue sensitivity to insulin.[216] Animal studies have indicated that vanadium may decrease blood glucose and improve insulin resistance.[213] Vanadium inhibits tyrosine phosphatase, thereby potentially upregulating tyrosine phosphorylation of the insulin receptor.[217]

Adverse Effects and Drug Interactions

Side effects of vanadium include diarrhea, abdominal cramping, nausea, and flatulence that may last a few days.[19] Greenish tongue discoloration has been reported, as well as fatigue and focal neurological lesions.[196] Serious safety issues have been raised from animal research, such as the potential for accumulation and subsequent toxicity.[218] Because vanadium inhibits tyrosine phosphatase, it may theoretically upregulate growth factor activity and thus work as a cancer promoter.[219, 220] Vanadium has been shown to accumulate in bone, but it also may be stored in the liver and kidneys and abnormal renal function has been associated with its use.[196, 213] Animal studies showed teratogenic effects.[124] Early reports intimated that excessive vanadium may be associated with bipolar disease.[221] Risks of long-term use are unknown.

Vanadium may potentiate the anticoagulant effects of antiplatelets.[222] Because it has digitalis-like effects in cardiac tissue, it may enhance therapeutic and/or adverse effects of digoxin.[19] Another theoretical interaction would be additive hypoglycemia with secretagogues.

Clinical Studies

Vanadium has been studied only in small numbers of humans and for a maximum period of a few weeks.[212] It has been studied in type 1 and type 2 diabetes. In a 2-week study, insulin dose decreased in patients with type 1 diabetes.[223] In a different single-blind, placebo-controlled study, six patients with type 2 diabetes were studied.[216] Patients took placebo for 2 weeks, then 50 mg twice daily of vanadyl sulfate for 3 weeks, and placebo again for 2 weeks. At the end of each treatment phase, a euglycemic hyperinsulinemic clamp and OGTT were done. Fasting plasma glucose declined from a baseline of 210 mg/dl (11.7 mmol/l) to 180 mg/dl (10.0 mmol/l; $P < 0.05$), and A1C declined from 9.6% to 8.8% ($P < 0.002$).

In another 4-week study of 8 patients with type 2 diabetes, 50 mg twice daily of vanadyl sulfate was administered in a single-blind, placebo-controlled study.[224] Six patients continued on placebo for an additional 4 weeks. Baseline euglycemic hyperinsulinemic clamps were done and then redone at the end of the treatment phase. Fasting glucose decreased significantly from 167 mg/dl (9.3 mmol/l) to 133 mg/dl (7.4 mmol/l; $P < 0.05$).

In 16 patients with type 2 diabetes, vanadyl sulfate was given at three different doses (75, 150, and 300 mg/day) for 6 weeks.[225] Fasting glucose decreased significantly only in the 300-mg group, from 167 mg/dl (9.3 mmol/l) at baseline to 144 mg/dl (8.0 mmol/l) at end point ($P < 0.02$). A1C decreased from 7.8% to 6.8% in the 150-mg group ($P < 0.05$) and from 7.1% to 6.8% in the 300-mg group ($P = 0.05$).

Summary

Although many people with diabetes use vanadium supplements, it has only been evaluated in a small number of individuals. It is estimated that fewer than 40 people have been involved in short-term studies.[19] Vanadium is a trace element found in grains and vegetables. Because of teratogenicity in animal studies, vanadium supplements are contraindicated in pregnant women. There is no established recommended daily allowance. The estimate of tolerable upper level for adults is 1.8 mg/day;[196] yet studies used doses far exceeding this amount (100–125 mg/day). Improvements included decreased fasting plasma glucose and A1C levels, decreased insulin requirements in patients with type 1 diabetes, and enhanced insulin sensitivity in patients with type 2 diabetes.[216, 223–225] Vanadium is a substance with great potential for toxicity, and vanadium supplementation is definitely not recommended.

NICOTINAMIDE

Nicotinamide is one form of vitamin B_3,[19] which is necessary for appropriate functioning of over 50 enzymes in the body. Nicotinamide is necessary to release energy, manufacture fats from carbohydrates, and synthesize sex hormones. Dietary sources of nicotinamide include fish, beans, yeast, bran, almonds, peanuts, wild or brown rice, whole wheat, barley, and peas.[19]

Nicotinamide has been used for a variety of conditions. These include peripheral vascular disease, pellagra, premenstrual headaches and migraines, cognitive impairment, bullous pemphigoid, and, in a topical form, acne.[19] The vitamin is available in two major forms: nicotinic acid (niacin) and nicotinamide (niacinamide). Both forms have similar effects in low doses. In high doses, they have differing effects: nicotinic acid is used as a treatment for dyslipidemia, and nicotinamide for diabetes and diabetes prevention.[19] Nicotinamide has been studied not only in diabetes prevention,[226] but also has been used to improve blood glucose control.[227, 228]

Mechanism of Action

Nicotinamide may preserve, improve, and protect β-cell function by improving resistance to autoimmune destruction. Nicotinamide is water soluble and is a precursor of nicotinamide adenine dinucleotide (NAD) and nicotinamide adenine dinucleotide phosphate (NADP), which are essential for oxidation-reduction synthesis, ADP ribose transfer reactions, and ATP synthesis.[19] Intracellularly, nicotinamide may inhibit the enzyme poly (ADP-ribose) polymerase (PARP), thereby preventing depletion of NAD^+. Low intracellular NAD^+ levels may contribute to islet cell destruction via apoptosis.[229]

Adverse Effects and Drug Interactions

Nicotinamide use may lead to skin reactions, headache, allergies, dizziness, nausea and vomiting, and diarrhea. Other adverse effects include blurry vision, hepatotoxicity, hypoalbuminemia, and abnormal prothrombin times. Nicotinamide use warrants monitoring liver enzymes, platelet function, and blood glucose.[19] Use is contraindicated in patients with active liver disease. Nicotinamide may exacerbate gallbladder disease, gout, peptic ulcer disease, and allergies. There is a potential for decreased insulin sensitivity and decreased first-phase insulin release.

Nicotinamide may increase serum drug concentrations of certain anticonvulsants, such as primidone or carbamazepine.[230] Combination with chronic heavy alcohol use or hepatotoxic drugs or CAM supplements (such as kava, comfrey, or pennyroyal) may lead to liver toxicity. Concomitant use with secretagogues may result in additive hypoglycemia.

Clinical Studies

Nicotinamide trials in diabetes have focused on prevention and treatment. A large prevention trial was conducted in high-risk children in New Zealand.[226] Islet cell antibodies (ICAs) were measured in over 20,000 children. A total of 185 children had positive ICA levels, and 173 received 500 mg twice daily of nicotinamide. Average follow-up time was 7.1 years. The incidence of diabetes was 60% lower in children given nicotinamide.

A long-term randomized, double-blind, placebo-controlled trial, the European Nicotinamide Diabetes Intervention Trial (ENDIT), evaluated whether regular use of nicotinamide can prevent diabetes.[231] This study included 549 subjects who had a first-degree family member with type 1 diabetes and had positive islet cell antibodies. Patients were given 1.2 g/m^2 of modified-release nicotinamide or placebo for 5 years. A total of 159 subjects developed diabetes; 82 were on nicotinamide and 77 were on placebo ($P = 0.69$).

A meta-analysis of 10 randomized trials in 211 recently diagnosed patients with type 1 diabetes reported higher C-peptide levels in nicotinamide-treated patients than in the placebo group after 1 year of treatment.[227] There were no significant differences in insulin doses or A1C levels after 1 year. A 6-month single-blind trial in 18 patients with type 2 diabetes reported improved C-peptide levels in the groups receiving nicotinamide.[228] Another 2-year trial in 64 children with recent-onset type 1 diabetes found that nicotinamide (25 mg/kg/day) alone or combined with vitamin E (15 mg/kg/day) along with intensive insulin treatment preserved C-peptide levels at 2 years.[232] There was no difference between the groups in A1C. The same group of researchers did a retrospective analysis and compared 25 children in whom nicotinamide (25 mg/kg/day) was added to intensive insulin therapy at diagnosis with a group of 27 children who were only on intensive insulin therapy.[233] After 2 years, A1C was lower in the insulin-plus-nicotinamide group than in the insulin-only group (6.09% vs. 6.98%, respectively, $P < 0.01$).

Summary

Nicotinamide is a B vitamin that has been used for diabetes prevention and treatment. It is not a benign substance, and varying adverse effects and drug interactions, especially with hepatotoxic agents, may occur. Although varying results have been obtained, the definitive trial, ENDIT, has determined that nicotinamide is not effective in preventing type 1 diabetes. Although nicotinamide may help somewhat in diabetes control, the results are not definitive and patients should be warned that long-term study is warranted. Doses used have ranged in studies, based on surface area or weight (25 mg/kg/day), and in an early trial, the dose used was 500 mg twice daily. Nicotinamide use should be discouraged until long-term trial results and more information are obtained.

MAGNESIUM

Magnesium is one of the most abundant cations in the body and is used medically as an antacid and for many different conditions such as constipation, preeclampsia, pregnancy-related leg cramps, various cardiovascular diseases including hypertension and arrhythmias, migraine headaches, and diabetes.[19] Dietary sources of magnesium include green leafy vegetables, legumes, grains, seeds, nuts, meats, coffee, and dark chocolate.[234–237]

It has been estimated that 25%–38% of people with type 2 diabetes may have hypomagnesemia and that supplementation may improve diabetes control.[238] Furthermore, hypomagnesemia has been theorized as being associated with diabetes-related complications such as neuropathy[238] and foot ulcers.[239]

Mechanism of Action

Magnesium is available in numerous forms, such as sulfate, citrate, hydroxide, oxide, and chloride salts. Magnesium is a cofactor for different enzymes in different glucose metabolic pathways and phosphorylation reactions.[235, 240] Magnesium deficiency may be a factor in several disease states, including diabetes. Low dietary magnesium consumption may play a role in insulin resistance and development of type 2 diabetes.[19] With hypomagnesemia there is diminished insulin action and potential insulin resistance related to reduced tyrosine kinase activity at the insulin receptor and possibly resultant impaired insulin action caused by impaired insulin signaling.[234, 240, 241]

Adverse Effects and Drug Interactions

Adverse effects include gastrointestinal irritation, nausea, vomiting, and diarrhea, as well as hypermagnesemia when given to patients with diminished renal function.[19] Numerous drugs, including diuretics, digoxin, beta-2 agonists, steroids, cyclosporine, and several others, may deplete magnesium. Magnesium use may result in additive hypotension with concomitant calcium-channel blocker use or result in hypermagnesemia if used with potassium-sparing diuretics such as spironolactone. When administered concomitantly, magnesium may impair absorption of certain drugs such as tetracyclines, fluoroquinolones, calcium products, and bisphosphonates.[19]

Clinical Studies

Magnesium intake and risk of type 2 diabetes has been evaluated with varying results. One prospective study in over 12,000 individuals assessed low magnesium levels as well as magnesium intake and risk of diabetes.[240] The study found there was no association between dietary magnesium consumption and risk of type 2 diabetes, but also found that low serum magnesium level was predictive of developing type 2 diabetes. A different study conducted food-frequency questionnaires every 2–4 years in a large group of individuals (85,060 women and 42,872 men) followed for 12 or 18 years (men and women, respectively). In this study, the investigators found that low dietary magnesium intake was correlated with increased diabetes risk.[235]

Studies evaluating magnesium use in established diabetes range from showing no effect to showing potential benefit. One study that describes benefits of oral magnesium supplementation in type 2 diabetes was a 16-week randomized, double-blind, placebo-controlled trial in 63 patients with decreased magnesium concentrations who were taking a sulfonylurea.[241] Thirty-two patients were supplemented daily with 50 ml magnesium chloride solution (50 g magnesium chloride per 1,000 ml solution), and 31 took placebo. The patients in the treatment group had decreased mean fasting glucose and A1C after 16 weeks, from 230 mg/dl (12.8 mmol/l) to 144 mg/dl (8.0 mmol/l) and from 11.5% to 8%, respectively ($P < 0.05$ for both). Those in the control group also had significant declines, from 256 mg/dl (14.2 mmol/l) to 185 mg/dl

(10.3 mmol/l) and from 11.8% to 10.1% ($P < 0.05$ for both). There was a significant difference favoring the treatment group ($P < 0.05$ for fasting glucose and A1C). A measure of insulin sensitivity, the HOMA-IR (homeostasis model assessment of insulin resistance) index, also improved in the treatment group (4.3 at baseline and 3.8 at treatment end, $P < 0.05$) but not in the control group (4.7 at baseline and 5.0 at study end).

One study that describes equivocal benefit was a 30-day randomized, double-blind, placebo-controlled study using two different doses of magnesium or placebo for 30 days in 128 patients with type 2 diabetes.[238] A total of 47.7% of the patients had hypomagnesemia. Magnesium oxide (20.7 mmol or 41.4 mmol) was administered daily. Plasma glucose increased nonsignificantly in the treatment groups, from 185 mg/dl (10.3 mmol/l) at baseline to 207 mg/dl (11.5 mmol/l) at study end in the lower-dose group and from 227 mg/dl (12.6 mmol/l) at baseline to 229 mg/dl (12.7 mmol/l) at study end in the higher-dose group. A1C decreased nonsignificantly in the lower-dose group (10.2% to 9.7% at study end) and increased nonsignificantly in the higher-dose group (9.0% at baseline to 9.2% at study end). However, fructosamine declined significantly in the higher-dose group (4.1 mmol/l at baseline and 3.75 mmol/l at study end, $P < 0.05$).

A study that showed no change in metabolic control was done in 40 people with type 2 diabetes.[242] The patients had low magnesium levels and were given magnesium citrate (30 mmol/day) for 3 months. A1C increased slightly, but the change was not significant (7.2% at baseline and 7.4% at study end). In insulin-requiring type 2 patients, a different study also showed no improvement in metabolic parameters.[243] A total of 50 patients were administered 15 mmol/day magnesium aspartate hydrochloride or placebo for 3 months. There was no difference in plasma glucose between the treatment and control groups at study end (193 mg/dl [10.7 mmol/l] vs. 209 mg/dl [11.6 mmol/l], respectively; $P = 0.8$), although glucose declined nonsignificantly in the treatment group (212 mg/dl [11.8 mmol/l] at baseline to 193 mg/dl [10.7 mmol//l] at study end). A1C did not differ in the treatment and control groups (8.9% vs. 9.1%, $P = 0.6$).

Summary

Magnesium deficiency may result in predisposition to type 2 diabetes or, in those with established type 2 diabetes, diminished metabolic control. However, there are no clear-cut guidelines on when to assess whether a person may have magnesium deficiency, unless he or she is taking certain medications or has a disease that may deplete magnesium. Magnesium-depleting medications may include certain diuretics, steroids, cyclosporine, tacrolimus, digoxin, beta-2 agonists, and aminoglycosides. Magnesium supplementation is controversial at best, and it is difficult to determine which patients would benefit; therefore, periodic testing for hypomagnesemia may be done at least annually. There is a fine line between repletion of magnesium and magnesium toxicity. Certain patient groups, such as those with impaired renal function, should not take magnesium supplements because of the kidneys' inability to adequately clear the magnesium.

The longest study thus far that favors magnesium supplementation was a 16-week trial in which the daily dose was 50 ml magnesium chloride solution (containing 50 g/1,000 ml of solution).[241] Use beyond 4 months has not been documented. The ADA consensus statement on magnesium[244] indicates that prospective long-term studies are needed to determine whether hypomagnesemia predisposes patients to complication risks and that baseline serum magnesium concentrations should be determined in certain disease states associated with hypomagnesemia, such as congestive heart failure (CHF) or coronary artery disease, long-term parenteral nutrition, pregnancy, or ethanol abuse. Many studies differ as to the benefit of magnesium supplementation and the type of magnesium salt, dose, and duration of treatment. The tolerable upper intake dose from supplements and pharmacological agents in addition to magnesium intake from food and water is 350 mg daily and higher doses may result in diarrhea.[19] Overall, chronic magnesium supplementation is not recommended at this time.

COENZYME Q10

Coenzyme Q10 (CoQ10) is also known as ubiquinone because it is found in almost all human cells. It is a lipid-soluble, vitamin-like substance. Humans synthesize CoQ10, and it is highly concentrated in the brain, heart, liver, kidneys, and pancreas.[19, 245] Dietary sources of CoQ10 include poultry, beef, and broccoli, but dietary supplements are manufactured via beet and sugarcane fermentation with special yeast strains.[19, 246] CoQ10 levels decline with age and with the presence of certain disease states, such as CHF, cardiomyopathy, hypertension, Parkinson's disease, cancer, and periodontal disease.[247]

CoQ10 has been used as adjunctive therapy for various cardiac diseases, including CHF and hypertension, Parkinson's disease, cancer, muscular dystrophy, and periodontal disease.[19, 245] There is preliminary evidence that it may be useful in treating diabetes.[248]

Chemical Constituents and Mechanism of Action

CoQ10 has a 10-carbon side chain (hence the name), and its structure is similar to that of vitamin K.[19, 245] The primary biochemical activity is as a cofactor in the electron transport chain involved in mitochondrial ATP production. CoQ10 may function as a direct membrane stabilizer, secondary to phospholipid-protein interactions. It may serve as an antioxidant and free-radical scavenger. Oxygen-derived free radicals may inactivate endothelium-derived relaxing factor, which may result in arteriolar constriction. Ischemic tissues may also have oxygen-derived free radicals, and CoQ10 may be protective in tissues where these oxygen-derived free radicals may exert damage.[19, 245] In diabetes, it is theorized that there may be suboptimal CoQ10 activity in β-cells and that by increasing activity of glycerol-3-phosphate dehydrogenase and improving ATP production, CoQ10 may improve glucose-stimulated insulin secretion.[249]

Adverse Effects and Drug Interactions

In a few patients, gastric upset, including diarrhea, nausea, anorexia, and epigastric distress, has occurred. Although early reports stated there were dose-related increases in serum glutamic oxaloacetic transaminase, long-term administration of 600 mg/day has not changed liver function.[19] Long-term administration for 6 years has not resulted in any adverse effects.[250]

Since CoQ10 is a structural analog to vitamin K, it may decrease INR when combined with warfarin, although a prospective trial showed that 4 weeks of concomitant use did not result in decreased INR.[251] Smoking depletes CoQ10 levels.[19] A controversial drug interaction is that treatment with statins may decrease endogenous levels of CoQ10 and that this may be a mechanism responsible for statin-related myopathy.[252] A crossover study that used lower doses of pravastatin and atorvastatin did not result in lower CoQ10 levels,[253] but another study also using low atorvastatin doses[254] and higher doses [255] did find depletion of CoQ10. Decreased CoQ10 concentrations with statin treatment have also been reported in patients with diabetes.[256] Additive hypotension with antihypertensives may occur, as well as additive effects on hypoglycemia if combined with secretagogues. A potentially beneficial drug interaction has occurred with doxorubicin. CoQ10 supplementation may diminish doxorubicin-mediated cardiotoxicity[257] by thwarting inhibition of CoQ10 enzymes.

Clinical Studies

Coenzyme Q10 has been evaluated extensively in cardiac disease. In a study of 109 patients with hypertension, CoQ10 administration was added to existing treatment with antihypertensive agents.[258] There were no details of blinding, and there was no comparison group. The dose of CoQ10 was adjusted to maintain a blood level of 2.0 μg/ml; the average dose was 225 mg/day. Patients were followed for an average of 13 months. Mean systolic pressure decreased from 159 mmHg to 147 mmHg

($P < 0.001$), and mean diastolic pressure decreased from 94 mmHg to 85 mmHg ($P < 0.001$).

In a randomized, double-blind trial of hypertensive patients, 30 patients received 60 mg CoQ10 twice a day and 30 patients received a vitamin B complex for 8 weeks.[259] Mean blood pressure decreased from 168 mmHg to 152 mmHg systolic and 106 mmHg to 97 mmHg diastolic in the patients treated with CoQ10 ($P < 0.05$ vs. baseline); whereas the patients on the vitamin B complex went from mean baseline systolic blood pressure of 166 mmHg to 164 mmHg and from mean baseline diastolic blood pressure of 105 mmHg to 103 mmHg at end point (P not significant). The difference between groups was significant, favoring CoQ10 ($P < 0.05$). Although the authors reported subjects were not diagnosed with diabetes, patients were thought to have insulin resistance, and mean baseline glucose decreased in the CoQ10 group from 141 mg/dl (7.8 mmol/l) to 95 mg/dl (5.3 mmol/l) at 8 weeks ($P < 0.05$ vs. baseline). Mean baseline declines in the vitamin B complex–treated group were not significant (140 mg/dl [7.8 mmol/l] vs. 129 mg/dl [7.2 mmol/l], respectively). Mean fasting plasma insulin decreased from 465 pmol/l to 257 pmol/l in the CoQ10 group ($P < 0.05$ vs. baseline). This did not change significantly in the vitamin B–complex group.

For CHF, the data is controversial. In general, CoQ10 has improved number of hospitalizations and certain clinical parameters such as edema and dyspnea. In a 1-year randomized, double-blind, placebo-controlled trial of 641 patients with heart failure, there were fewer hospitalizations for heart failure and fewer episodes of pulmonary edema.[260] However, a recent study with excellent study design and well-defined parameters found no benefit with CoQ10 in 55 patients with New York Heart Association class III and IV symptoms.[261] In this trial, CoQ10 administration did not benefit ejection fraction, peak oxygen consumption, or exercise duration in patients with CHF receiving standard medical therapy. An ongoing long-term outcome trial with over 500 people with New York Heart Association class III and IV CHF who will be followed for over 2 years will hopefully better define the role of CoQ10 in CHF.[262]

In a randomized, double-blind, placebo-controlled trial, 34 patients with type 1 diabetes were administered 100 mg/day CoQ10 or placebo for 3 months.[263] A1C decreased from 8.04% to 7.86% in the CoQ10 group and from 8.02% to 7.84% in the placebo group. Differences from baseline and between groups were not significant. Mean daily blood glucose decreased from 160 mg/dl (8.9 mmol/l) at baseline to 145 mg/dl (8.1 mmol/l) in the CoQ10 group and from 161 mg/dl (8.9 mmol/l) at baseline to 153 mg/dl (8.5 mmol/l) in the placebo group. Differences from baseline and between groups were not significant. Insulin doses did not change in either group. There were no significant differences in systolic or diastolic blood pressures from baseline in either group. Differences between groups were also not significant.

Another 6-month randomized, placebo-controlled trial in 23 patients with type 2 diabetes on sulfonylureas assessed metabolic control when 100 mg twice daily of CoQ10 was administered.[264] Although CoQ10 administration resulted in a greater than threefold increase in serum concentration, there was no improvement in diabetes control. Mean baseline A1C increased from baseline 8.1% to 9.1% at 6 months in the CoQ10 group and from 7.9% to 8.1% in the placebo group (*P* values not reported). Fasting glucose decreased from a baseline of 211 mg/dl (11.7 mmol/l) to 198 mg/dl (11.0 mmol/l) in the CoQ10 group and from 203 mg/dl (11.3 mmol/l) to 191 mg/dl (10.6 mmol/l) in the placebo group (*P* values not reported).

Another randomized, controlled trial assessed the effect of CoQ10 administration on blood glucose and blood pressure in 74 patients with type 2 diabetes and dyslipidemia.[265] Patients were randomized to 100 mg CoQ10 twice daily or 200 mg fenofibrate daily, combination of CoQ10 and fenofibrate, or placebo for 12 weeks. The authors reported *P* values for main effects of CoQ10 and fenofibrate as between-group differences in postintervention values after adjusting for baseline values; they also stated that there was no significant interaction for any variables in the fenofibrate-plus-CoQ10 arm and were thus not included in the numbers. It is difficult to analyze the statistical methods because the

CoQ10 group went from a baseline A1C of 6.9% to 7% at end point and the combination (CoQ10 plus fenofibrate) group went from baseline A1C of 7.5% to 7.2%. Yet the authors reported A1C decreased significantly, by 0.37% ($P = 0.032$) in the CoQ10 group. The combination group may have benefited from the impact of fenofibrate on triglyceride lowering. The authors also reported that systolic pressure declined by 6.1 mmHg ($P = 0.021$) and diastolic pressure decreased by 2.9 mmHg ($P = 0.048$) with CoQ10 supplementation.

Summary

CoQ10 is a vitamin-like substance that has been studied for a variety of cardiovascular disorders as well as for diabetes. One of the most unique reasons CoQ10 has been used by people with hyperlipidemia is that there may be statin-associated decreased serum CoQ10 concentrations, that may lead to myopathy. However, this benefit has not been conclusively shown.[19, 245] Adverse effects have been rare even with long-term use. Patients should be warned that INR might decrease if they are on warfarin and that possible additive hypotension or hypoglycemia may occur if the patient is on antihypertensives or secretagogues, respectively. Although CoQ10 is a much-studied agent for cardiovascular disease, many studies have used an open-label study design, which may result in unintentional bias. Other studies have not used a control group. In still other trials, study design has been inadequate (lacking randomization or blinding) and end points have not always been acceptable or well defined. The hypertension studies, for example, had an unacceptable end point. Although systolic and diastolic blood pressures decreased significantly, end point pressures were still much higher than would be advocated for a patient with diabetes. In studies of patients with type 1 or type 2 diabetes, CoQ10 supplementation has shown neutral to slightly improved effects on fasting glucose and A1C. Doses have varied in different studies. For hypertension and other cardiovascular diseases, the dose has ranged from 100 mg/day to 225 mg/day, although up to 600 mg in divided doses has been used for varying cardiovascular diseases.[19] In diabetes, the dose is 100–200 mg/day.[263–265] Even though there is much enthusiasm for CoQ10 and long-term studies have not shown harmful effects, further long-term studies are needed to determine its place in therapy.

Table 2. Nonbotanical CAM Supplements Used to Treat Diabetes

Nonbotanical Product	Chemical Constituents	Mechanism of Action	Side Effects & Drug Interactions
Chromium	Trivalent chromium [19,75]	• May enhance cellular effects of insulin through enhanced tyrosine kinase activity • May ↑ number of insulin receptors • May ↑ insulin binding or insulin activation [191,193]	*Side effects:* • Related to excessive intake and include renal toxicity, thrombocytopenia, hepatic dysfunction, rhabdomyolysis [193,197,198,199] • Dermatologic reactions [200] *Drug interactions:* • May ↓ blood glucose if used with secretagogues [19] • Some drugs ↓ chromium (steroids, acid blockers) [19] • Some drugs ↑ chromium (vitamin C, NSAIDs) [19]
Vanadium	Trace element [19,212]	• May function in various parts of the insulin-signaling pathway • May have insulin-mimetic activity and ↑ tissue sensitivity to insulin [213,215,216]	*Side effects:* • GI upset [19] • Animal research shows potential for accumulation [196,213] • Green tongue discoloration [19,196]

(Continued)

Table 2. (*Continued*)

Nonbotanical Product	Chemical Constituents	Mechanism of Action	Side Effects & Drug Interactions
		• Inhibits tyrosine phosphatase thereby upregulating insulin receptor tyrosine phosphorylation [217]	• May work as cancer promoter [219,220] • Per animal data, teratogenic effects [124] • Possible association with bipolar disease [221] *Drug interactions:* • May potentiate anticoagulant effects of antiplatelet agents [222] • May potentiate therapeutic or toxic effects of digoxin [19,75]
Nicotinamide	Vitamin B$_3$ [19,75]	• May improve and preserve β-cell function • May inhibit an enzyme (poly[ADP-ribose]polymerase or PARP) responsible for depletion of NAD$^+$, thereby preventing islet cell destruction via apoptosis [19,229]	*Side effects:* • Headache • Skin reactions, allergies • GI upset • May trigger gout and peptic ulcer disease • May adversely affect liver function—monitor liver function tests and platelet function [19,75]

Drug interactions:
- May ↑ serum concentrations of certain anticonvulsants (carbamazepine, primidone) [230]
- Liver toxicity if heavy alcohol use [19]
- Possible additive hypoglycemia if used with secretagogues [19]

Magnesium	• Numerous salt forms - sulfate - citrate - hydroxide - oxide - chloride [235]	• Cofactor for enzymes in glucose metabolic pathways and phosphorylation reactions [235,240] • Low dietary magnesium may contribute to insulin resistance and ↓ insulin action [19,234,240,241]

Side effects:
- GI upset
- Hypermagnesemia and magnesium accumulation in renal disease [19]

Drug interactions:
- May impair absorption of certain antibiotics, calcium, bisphosphonates
- Additive hypotension with calcium blockers
- Hypermagnesemia with potassium sparing diuretics

(*Continued*)

Table 2. (*Continued*)

Nonbotanical Product	Chemical Constituents	Mechanism of Action	Side Effects & Drug Interactions
			• Many drugs deplete magnesium (diuretics, steroids, beta-2 agonists, digoxin, cyclosporine) [19]
Coenzyme Q10	• 10-carbon side chain with similar structure to vitamin K [19,245]	• Antioxidant • Membrane stabilizer • Cofactor in metabolism in ATP production and oxidative respiration [19,245] • ↑ glycerol-3-phosphate dehydrogenase activity thus improving glucose-stimulated insulin secretion [249]	*Side effects:* • GI upset • No serious effects seen with long-term use [19,250] *Drug interactions:* • Theoretical additive hypoglycemia if combined with secretagogues [19] • May antagonize effects of warfarin and ↓ INR [251] • Statins may lower CoQ10 levels [252–256] • Additive hypotension with antihypertensives [19] • ↓ cardiotoxicity of doxorubicin [257]

4.

Botanical and Nonbotanical CAM Supplements that May Treat Complications of Diabetes

Complications of diabetes may be devastating and disruptive to patients' lives. Many individuals search for CAM supplements in the hope of preventing or treating diabetes-related complications. These supplements include both botanical and nonbotanical products, and they have varying actions and pharmacological profiles. Table 3 (on page 146) provides a brief summary of the information in this section.

ALPHA-LIPOIC ACID

Alpha-lipoic acid (ALA), also known as thioctic acid, is a disulfide compound synthesized in the liver. ALA functions similarly to B-complex vitamins in the body, and dietary sources include broccoli, spinach, potatoes, yeast, and liver.[75] ALA is a catalytic agent associated with pyruvate dehydrogenase. In carbohydrate metabolism in vivo, ALA functions as a cofactor and interacts with pyrophosphatase to convert pyruvic acid to acetyl-coenzyme A (in the Krebs cycle) and to produce energy in the form of adenosine triphosphate.[19, 266] ALA may increase insulin sensitivity.[267]

ALA has been used in Germany to treat peripheral neuropathy.[19] Other clinical applications include potential uses in ischemic reperfusion injury, cataracts, glaucoma, and *Amanita phalloides* poisoning. Other potential targets include neurological disorders such as Parkinson's and Alzheimer's disease.[266]

Chemical Constituents and Mechanism of Action

ALA is readily converted to the reduced form dihydrolipoic acid (DHLA). ALA and DHLA are both potent antioxidants and act as free-radical scavengers.[267, 268] Both ALA and DHLA help regenerate endogenous antioxidants, including vitamins C and E and glutathione. Because it can chelate metals and scavenge free radicals, ALA is considered an ideal antioxidant.

In people with diabetes, indirect markers of oxidative stress, such as malondialdehyde and 8-hydroxydeoxyguanosine levels, are increased.[269] Other oxidative-stress markers that are increased in diabetes include superoxide anion and peroxynitrite, as well as increased levels of vascular dysfunction markers such as nuclear factor-κB and thrombomodulin.[270] These markers of oxidative stress and other markers are implicated in the pathogenesis of diabetic neuropathy.[269] Since ALA may decrease oxidative stress and improve impaired microcirculation, it may help to minimize symptoms of neuropathy.

In vitro, ALA stimulates translocation of glucose transporter systems (GLUT4) and increases glucose transport. It may also help protect against impaired insulin-stimulated protein kinase B activation.[271]

Adverse Effects and Drug Interactions

To date, no serious side effects from ALA have been reported, even though it has been used intravenously and in long-term trials.[272–274] However, ALA may produce dose-related gastrointestinal side effects, including nausea and vomiting, as well as vertigo.[275] Allergic skin conditions are also possible. Anecdotal information indicates that ALA may lower triiodothyroxine levels, therefore thyroid function should be monitored.[19]

Hypoglycemia may occur when ALA is combined with secretago-gues.[268] Other theoretical interactions are related to mineral deficiency, since ALA is a chelating agent. Because animal research has shown ALA to produce toxicity in thiamine-deficiency, supplementation with vitamin B should be considered in individuals who abuse alcohol and therefore may be thiamine deficient. Since antacids may bind ALA, administration should be spaced at least a few hours apart.[19]

Clinical Studies

ALA has been studied in a series of Alpha-Lipoic Acid in Diabetic Neu-ropathy (ALADIN) trials. The first ALADIN trial was a randomized, double-blind, placebo-controlled trial in 260 type 2 diabetes patients with symptomatic peripheral neuropathy.[272] Patients were given placebo or intravenous ALA (100, 600, or 1,200 mg/day). Total symptom scores decreased significantly for all three ALA doses versus placebo ($P < 0.05$). Burning, paresthesia, and numbness decreased significantly in patients on 600 and 1,200 mg versus placebo ($P < 0.05$). Pain scores decreased sig-nificantly only in the 600-mg versus placebo group ($P < 0.05$). The main decrease in Hamburg Pain Adjective List was significant for the 600- and 1,200-mg groups ($P < 0.01$). The neurodisability score, which measures vibration, pinprick, ankle reflexes, and temperature sensation in the great toe, decreased, but the decrease was significant only for the 1,200-mg group versus placebo ($P = 0.03$). A1C declined in all groups, but not significantly.

ALADIN II was a randomized, double-blind, placebo-controlled trial in 65 patients with type 1 or type 2 diabetes with polyneuropathy symptoms.[273] ALA (600 or 1,200 mg) or placebo was administered in-travenously for 5 days; then patients received 600 or 1,200 mg/day of ALA or placebo orally for 2 years. Mean sural nerve conduction velocity changes were significant for both doses of ALA versus placebo ($P < 0.05$). Sural sensory nerve action potential scores decreased significantly only in the 600-mg group, and tibial motor nerve conduction velocity changed significantly only in the 1,200-mg group ($P < 0.05$ for both parameters vs. placebo). Neurodisability score did not decrease, but the sample may have been too small to detect changes. Mean A1C decreases were not significant, although A1C decreased from 9.1% to 8% after 24 months in the 1,200-mg group.

ALADIN III was a randomized, double-blind, placebo-controlled trial in 503 patients with type 2 diabetes.[274] One group of patients received 600 mg of ALA intravenously for 3 weeks and then was randomized to 600 mg ALA three times daily orally or placebo orally for 6 months. The other group received intravenous placebo for 3 weeks, followed by oral placebo for 6 months. Mean baseline neuropathic impairment scores decreased after 19 days in the two ALA groups versus placebo ($P = 0.02$). However, after 7 months, differences were not significant between the groups. Mean A1C declines were also not significant.

The NATHAN I (Neurological Assessment of Thioctic Acid in Neuropathy) trial is an ongoing long-term, multicenter trial in North America and Europe that is assessing the role of ALA given orally in prevention and treatment of diabetes neuropathy.[276] NATHAN II addressed the use of an intravenous agent for relief of painful neuropathy symptoms, but this has not yet been published. The SYDNEY trial was a randomized controlled trial that evaluated 120 patients.[277] ALA or placebo was administered intravenously 5 days per week for a total of 14 treatments. Symptom scores declined significantly. A meta-analysis of 1,258 subjects in trials that used intravenous ALA or placebo (ALADIN I and III trials, the NATHAN II and SYDNEY trials) found that 52.7% of patients on ALA versus 36.9% on placebo had improved total symptom scores.[278] The 5-week multicenter, randomized, double-blind, placebo-controlled SYDNEY 2 trial evaluated three different doses of ALA (600 mg, 1,200 mg, and 1,800 mg) versus placebo in 181 patients with diabetes.[275] Total symptom scores declined significantly by 51%, 48%, and 52%, respectively, in the active treatment groups versus 32% in the placebo group ($P < 0.05$ vs. placebo). The response rates of $\geq 50\%$ in total symptom scores were 62%, 50%, 56%, and 26% in the ALA groups versus placebo ($P < 0.05$ vs. placebo).

Summary

ALA may benefit neuropathy secondary to diabetes because it is an antioxidant. However, there is no evidence that it prevents neuropathy. The clinical significance of reported improvements in neuropathy parameters in the ALADIN studies may be enhanced quality of life for patients with neuropathy. Although ALA has been used for several years in Germany, long-term trials are needed to determine whether ALA slows progression or only improves neuropathy symptoms. Decreases in A1C levels have not been significant.[272–274] Clinicians should monitor thyroid function tests, since ALA may decrease triiodothyroxine levels. Because ALA may produce toxicity in thiamine deficiency, clinicians should also consider whether patients taking ALA are candidates for thiamine supplementation in situations where thiamine deficiency may occur (as in alcohol abuse). Since ALA is a chelating agent, individuals who use antacids should space ALA doses a few hours apart. Typical doses of oral ALA have been 600–1,200 mg/day,[273, 274] although the recent SYDNEY 2 trial provides evidence for as little as 600 mg/day orally.[275] The SYDNEY 2 trial also showed that although pain improved significantly as part of the total symptom score, paresthesias and numbness did not improve. Although ALA is a benign agent, much is still unknown about its use.

VITAMIN E

Vitamin E is an essential fat-soluble vitamin necessary for human wellness. It is available as acetate, succinate, or other salts. Food sources include poultry, eggs, fruits, cereal grains, vegetables, vegetable oil, and wheat germ oil.[19, 75]

Vitamin E is used as a supplement and for treating or preventing a wide range of conditions and diseases, including aging, inflammatory skin disorders, cystic mastitis, malabsorption syndromes, cancer, Alzheimer's disease, Parkinson's disease, and many other disease states. It has also been used for intermittent claudication, neuropathy, cataracts, diabetes and its complications, as well as cardiovascular disease.[19, 75]

Chemical Constituents and Mechanism of Action

Vitamin E, or alpha-tocopherol, consists of eight stereoisomers. Also known as RRR-alpha-tocopherol, d-alpha-tocopherol has the greatest biologic activity and is called "natural" vitamin E. On the other hand, dl-alpha-tocopherol is the racemic mixture and more appropriately termed all-rac-alpha-tocopherol. The dl-alpha-tocopherol is also called "synthetic" vitamin E. It has less biologic activity than natural vitamin E.[279] Both natural and synthetic vitamin E are found in supplements, while the synthetic form is found in vitamin E–fortified foods.

Although deficiency does not result in a disease state, muscle weakness and erythrocyte viability are associated with low serum vitamin E concentrations. The mechanism of action is antioxidant activity to prevent free-radical formation.[279] Natural vitamin E is thought to have anti-inflammatory effects and thus possibly a benefit in atherosclerosis, but the mechanism has been difficult to determine. Oxidative metabolites may contribute to nephropathy; hence vitamin E may help slow renal disease progression.[280]

Adverse Effects and Drug Interactions

Adverse effects are unusual, but some events include gastrointestinal upset, weakness, headache, blurred vision, and rash. Adverse effects are associated with daily doses greater than 400 IU of either natural or synthetic vitamin E. Heart failure has been associated with vitamin E use.[281] One analysis noted that higher doses (> 150 IU/day) were associated with all-cause mortality.[282]

High-dose vitamin E has been associated with bleeding reactions due to interference with production of vitamin K–dependent clotting factors.[279, 283] Therefore, use of high-dose vitamin E with drugs or other CAM supplements that have antiplatelet activity should be avoided. An important interaction has been antagonism of the beneficial effect of statins on HDL cholesterol, resulting in HDL lowering.[284] There are many other possible interactions with other drugs or CAM supplements.[19] One interaction is decreased effects of vitamin K if vitamin E is used in high doses. Many substances may affect absorption of oil-soluble vitamins, including vitamin E, if taken at the same time. These include orlistat, mineral oil, or bile acid sequestrants. Some anticonvulsants may lower vitamin E levels, including phenytoin, carbamazepine, and phenobarbital.[19]

Clinical Studies

In diabetes, vitamin E has been shown in some studies to improve oxidative stress and insulin action, but there are few studies, involving small numbers of patients. Some studies have been positive, while others have been negative. In one positive study, vitamin E, given as 900 mg/day for 3 months, decreased fasting glucose, A1C, and triglycerides in 25 elderly subjects with type 2 diabetes.[285]

In cardiovascular disease, vitamin E is one of the most researched substances, and reported results have been conflicting. In the Alpha-Tocopherol, Beta Carotene Cancer Prevention study, 29,133 male smokers without coronary heart disease were randomized to 50 mg alpha-tocopherol, 20 mg beta-carotene, both, or two different placebos for 6.1 years.[286] Vitamin E use did not produce a significant change in cardiovascular disease risk, but there was a 50% increase in hemorrhagic stroke. A 1.5 year study of 2,002 individuals with coronary atherosclerosis who took 800 mg alpha-tocopherol daily (later decreased to 400 mg) showed a significant risk reduction of the composite end point of cardiovascular death and nonfatal myocardial infarction (MI), primarily due to decrease in nonfatal MI.[287] The GISSI study evaluated 11,324 people who had survived a recent MI in a 3-year trial in which subjects were given n-3 polyunsaturated fatty acids, 300 mg vitamin E, both agents, or either of 2 placebos.[288] The vitamin E group did not show a significant effect on the combined end point of death, nonfatal MI, or nonfatal stroke. In the Heart Outcomes Prevention Evaluation study, 400 IU vitamin E daily did not result in a decrease in number of heart attacks, strokes, or deaths from heart disease in a trial lasting 4.5 years and including 9,541 subjects, including many with diabetes.[289] In the famous Heart Protection Study, 20,536 individuals with coronary disease, other vascular disease, or diabetes were randomized to a combination antioxidant vitamin containing 600 mg vitamin E, simvastatin, both agents, or 2 placebos.[290] In the vitamin E group, there were no significant decreases in cardiovascular mortality or other cardiovascular disease incidence.

Several meta-analyses describing effects of vitamin E have been performed, and the results have invariably shown there is no overall cardiovascular benefit. Not only has lack of benefit been described, but also the possibility of great harm has emerged. A recent meta-analysis demonstrated increased mortality with use of vitamin E doses >150 IU daily.[282]

Summary

Vitamin E is a product that has enjoyed tremendous popularity for several decades. The National Health and Nutrition Examination Survey estimated that approximately 24 million people consumed daily vitamin E doses of ≥400 IU.[291] Recommended daily vitamin E intake is 15 mg daily from food. This is equivalent to 22 IU of natural vitamin E or 33 IU of synthetic vitamin E. The tolerable upper limit is 1,000 mg daily, and the conversion factor is different for supplements, such that this amount is equivalent to 1,500 IU of natural vitamin E and 1,100 IU of synthetic vitamin E.[19] Although vitamin E was originally thought to be of benefit in diabetes, it has not consistently shown improvement in clinical parameters such as blood glucose or A1C. There is anecdotal evidence that it may help with diabetes-related neuropathy.[19] The most popular use of vitamin E has been for cardiovascular disease prevention and treatment. However, several major trials and meta-analyses have shown there is no overall benefit. At this point the AHA does not sanction vitamin E dietary supplement consumption and instead promotes eating antioxidant-containing foods, such as grains, fruits, and vegetables.[292]

The primary form of vitamin E that has been used as a supplement includes the alpha-tocopherol family. However, recent attention has focused on gamma-tocopherol, the major form consumed in the typical U.S. diet.[293] Unlike alpha-tocopherol, gamma-tocopherol has not been included in U.S. dietary intake recommendations. However, it is commonly found in plant seeds, vegetable oils, and nuts and legumes, including walnuts, pecans, and peanuts. Although plasma gamma-tocopherol concentrations are approximately one-tenth of alpha-tocopherol levels, it has excellent antioxidant capacity and is more potent in trapping reactive nitrogen oxide species. Furthermore, gamma-tocopherol has greater anti-inflammatory activity than alpha-tocopherol, including inhibition of cyclooxygenase-2 (COX-2), and the metabolite has natriuretic effects.[294]

Alpha-tocopherol supplementation suppresses circulating levels of gamma-tocopherol. This effect has been one of many reasons speculated why alpha-tocopherol supplementation has not been shown to have beneficial effects in atherosclerosis trials. Hence, various researchers theorize that gamma-tocopherol is the beneficial vitamin E isoform. A take-home message for clinicians is that dietary supplements containing gamma-tocopherol are becoming increasingly popular. Clearly, research evaluating the use of gamma-tocopherol supplements in human subjects needs to be done to fully understand the role of vitamin E in diabetes.

GAMMA-LINOLENIC ACID

There are two main types of essential fatty acids. They are considered essential because they must be obtained from nutritional sources, since the body cannot manufacture them. Gamma-linolenic acid (GLA) is an omega-6 (n-6) essential fatty acid and is one of the two main essential fatty acids. The other main type of essential fatty acid is n-3 fatty acid, represented by fish oil. GLA is obtained from three sources: evening primrose oil, black currant seed oil, and borage oil. The main source of GLA is evening primrose oil, which is extracted from evening primrose (*Oenothera biennis*), a North American native plant. This wildflower is a yellow annual or biennial that grows from about 3–10 feet (1–3 meters) tall. The dry pod, or fruit, contains many small seeds and are the main source of GLA.[19, 75]

GLA is used as a nutritional supplement or as an ingredient in food products in many countries. It has been used to treat hyperlipidemia, mastitis, premenstrual syndrome, eczema, rheumatoid arthritis, and other disease states. In diabetes, it has been used to treat peripheral neuropathy.[19, 75]

Chemical Constituents and Mechanism of Action

GLA from evening primrose oil is used in human studies in diabetes. In the body, linoleic acid is converted to GLA. The enzyme delta-6-desaturase regulates the conversion.[295] Two other metabolites of GLA are dihomogammalinolenic acid and arachidonic acid, prostaglandin precursors that regulate the balance of platelet aggregation (through production of prostaglandin E1, or PGE1, thromboxane, and prostacyclin). Dihomogammalinolenic acid and arachidonic acid also maintain blood flow in small neural blood vessels. In essence, GLA is a PGE1 precursor. Linolenic acid conversion to GLA is thought to be impaired in neuropathy, secondary to problems with delta-6-desaturase, potentially leading to problems with nerve function.[295] Supplementation with GLA may alleviate these problems.[296, 297]

In diabetes, it is theorized that disturbances of essential fatty acids and prostaglandins may cause microvascular abnormalities leading to diminished blood flow and neural hypoxia.[295] GLA metabolites are important in maintaining nerve membrane structure, nerve blood flow, and nerve conduction.[298] An exogenous source of GLA would bypass the need for conversion of linoleic acid to GLA. Animal data has shown that diabetes-related neuropathy might be improved by GLA administration. Since A1C levels do not improve with GLA, the beneficial effects on symptoms of neuropathy are not secondary to blood glucose control.[296, 297]

Adverse Effects and Drug Interactions

Most adverse effects of GLA are mild and include headache and gastrointestinal effects such as bloating and loose stools.[19, 75] There are reports of prolonged bleeding time and seizures.[19, 75] There is the theoretical possibility of increased bleeding if GLA is combined with other drugs or CAM supplements that have antiplatelet properties, due to effects of GLA on thromboxane and prostaglandins. A precaution regarding use of GLA in combination with phenothiazines has been urged, since seizures may occur with this combination because both agents may lower the seizure threshold.[19, 75]

Clinical Studies

Clinical trials have evaluated GLA use in peripheral neuropathy in both type 1 and type 2 diabetes. A 6-month randomized, double-blind, placebo-controlled trial in 22 patients with type 1 and type 2 diabetes evaluated the effects of GLA on peripheral neuropathy.[296] Twelve patients received 360 mg/day of GLA and 10 patients received placebo. At the end of 6 months, there was improvement in neuropathy symptom scores ($P < 0.001$) as well as in other parameters, including median and peroneal nerve function measurements and ankle heat and cold threshold values. Although A1C declined from 9.1% to 8.7% the change was not significant.

Another study was a year-long, multicenter, randomized, double-blind, placebo-controlled trial in 111 patients with type 1 and type 2 diabetes.[297] Patients were given 480 mg GLA or placebo. The investigators evaluated neuropathy and reported significant improvements in 13 of 16 parameters. Significant improvements occurred in the following neurophysiological and thermal-sensitivity parameters: peroneal and median motor nerve conduction velocity ($P < 0.01$), extensor digitorium brevis and thenar compound muscle action potential ($P < 0.01$), sural and median sensory nerve action potential ($P < 0.02$ and $P < 0.001$, respectively), and wrist heat and cold threshold ($P < 0.01$ for both). Neurological parameters that significantly improved included the following: arm muscle strength and leg sensation ($P < 0.01$ for both), arm tendon reflex and sensation ($P < 0.02$ for both), and leg tendon reflex ($P < 0.05$). A1C did not improve, but an interesting finding was that GLA response was better in those patients whose baseline A1C was <10%.

A published abstract evaluated impact of GLA on vibratory perception threshold and different autonomic neuropathy parameters.[299] The study was a year-long, randomized, double-blind, placebo-controlled trial of 51 patients with type 1 or type 2 diabetes and neuropathy. They received 480 mg GLA daily or placebo. In this study, GLA did not improve autonomic neuropathy parameters or vibratory perception threshold.

Summary

GLA is an n-6 essential fatty acid that has been used to treat neuropathy because it may improve problematic nerve membrane structure, impulse conduction, and nerve blood flow. Since A1C does not improve with GLA use, benefit is not secondary to blood glucose control. However, in one study,[297] the response was enhanced in subjects with a lower initial A1C. Some sources have stated that it may take several months to see results with GLA. Doses of GLA used to treat neuropathy are 360–480 mg/day.[296, 297, 299] Although research looks promising and GLA is relatively benign, a definitive role for GLA in the treatment of neuropathic complications is unknown at this time.

GINKGO (*Gingko biloba* L.)

Gingko biloba, also known as the maidenhair tree or ginkgo, has a unique history. It is one of the world's oldest living tree species, dating back over 200 million years to Permian period fossils.[75] It is the lone survivor of the family Ginkgoaceae. The trees, which can grow to 125 feet (over 38 meters), have a bilobed, fan-shaped leaf. The ginkgo species is dioecious, and male trees that are over 20 years old produce spring blossoms, while adult female trees bear a fruit that falls in autumn. The inner seed is edible and is sold in Asian markets.[75] The ginkgo tree lives a long time, some trees as long as 1,000 years. Extracts from dried leaves of younger trees are used in complementary therapies. Gingko biloba is one of the most commonly used supplements in Germany, and it is widely used for cerebrovascular insufficiency and dementia.[300]

Ginkgo has a wide range of uses and has gained prominence for treatment of Alzheimer's or multi-infarct dementia, cerebral insufficiency, peripheral arterial disease, antidepressant-induced sexual dysfunction, chilblains (hand and foot swelling from cold exposure), vertigo and tinnitus, altitude sickness, and asthma.[75] Ginkgo may help with visual problems by increasing ocular blood flow and may benefit glaucoma and macular degeneration.[19, 301] In diabetes, gingko biloba may be useful for peripheral circulatory problems (such as intermittent claudication) and retinopathy. The effect on insulin resistance is currently being studied.

Chemical Constituents and Mechanism of Action

Active ingredients include flavonoids (ginkgo flavone glycosides) and terpenoids (ginkgolides and bilobalides).[300] The flavone glycosides include quercetin, kaempferol, and isorhamnetin. These are thought to have antioxidant activity and inhibit platelet aggregation. The ginkgolides, one of the chemical constituents of terpenoids, are thought to improve circulation and inhibit platelet-activating factor. The bilobalides, the other constituents of the terpenoids, are thought to have neuroprotective properties.[19, 75, 300] Clinical studies have been done with products containing 24% flavone glycosides and 6% terpene lactones.[19]

Adverse Effects and Drug Interactions

Side effects have been varied. In fewer than 1% of patients, gastrointestinal upset may occur. Transient headache for the first 2–3 days has been reported with gingko biloba use. Exposure to the fruit pulp may result in cross-allergic reactions with members of the *Rhus* species (poison ivy). Eating the seed may result in seizures, due to the ginkgotoxin content.[19, 75] Providers should note that concomitant use of ginkgo with drugs that lower seizure threshold should be avoided.

Some of the most worrisome effects have been bleeding reactions, including subdural hematoma, subarachnoid hemorrhage, hyphema (bleeding from the margin of the iris), and retrobulbar hemorrhage. A recent review of case reports concluded that there may be a causal association of increased bleeding with ginkgo use and that further study is warranted.[302]

The main drug interaction is the potential for additive antiplatelet activity when combined with antiplatelet drugs, such as warfarin, aspirin, or Cox-2 inhibitors such as celecoxib, or with botanical products that also have antiplatelet activity, such as ginger, garlic, and feverfew.[19, 75] A case report indicated that concomitant use with a widely used antidepressant, trazodone, resulted in coma in a patient with dementia.[303] Also, an interaction involving a 17% decrease in alprazolam serum concentrations has been reported.[304]

Emerging evidence has shown that ginkgo may inhibit metabolism of drugs that are metabolized by various CYP450 isoenzymes, including 2D6, 1A2, and 2C9.[19] However, there are varying reports on the degree of enzyme inhibition, depending on in vitro or in vivo evaluation, and the clinical significance is not yet determined. Clinicians should therefore monitor the effects of certain medications and look for slightly increased blood levels of some antipsychotics and cardiac medications, caffeine, and warfarin. In addition, certain sulfonylureas are metabolized through 2C9, including glipizide and glyburide, so a theoretical potentiation of these drugs may occur. Effects on CYP 3A4 are variable, with some reports that indicate inhibition and others that indicate induction.[19]

Clinical Studies

The effect of 120 mg/day ginkgo for 3 months has been evaluated in three different studies that evaluated insulin secretion. In individuals with normal glucose, there was an increase in pancreatic insulin and C-peptide response measured as area under the curve during a 75-g OGTT.[305] In individuals with diet-controlled type 2 diabetes, there was no effect on insulin area under the curve with ginkgo. In the same study, however, gingko administration in type 2 diabetes patients on secretagogues resulted in altered insulin secretion and subsequent elevated blood glucose.[306] A recent report indicates that in a crossover comparison of ginkgo and placebo for

3 months in normal, pre-diabetes, and type 2 diabetes patients, there was no difference in glucose metabolic rates at low or high insulin infusion rates.[307]

Several studies have evaluated ginkgo in intermittent claudication and found that ginkgo may increase pain-free walking distance. In a 24-week randomized, double-blind, placebo-controlled trial in 111 patients, the subjects were initially able to walk only a short distance without pain.[308] Those who took 120 mg/day of ginkgo were able to improve pain-free walking distance by 40%, compared with 20% for the placebo group. Differences in maximum walking distance and relative increase of pain-free walking distance were significant ($P < 0.05$). A meta-analysis of eight studies of gingko in intermittent claudication reported an increase in pain-free walking distance.[309] Weighted mean difference with gingko was 34 meters (over 37 yards; 95% CI, 26–43 meters). Another analysis of nine studies with good study design (double-blind, placebo-controlled trials) was also done.[310] The trials evaluated 619 people taking 120–160 mg/day for 6–24 weeks. Results favored the ginkgo group.

A 3-month open-label study was conducted in 25 patients with type 2 diabetes and retinopathy.[311] The study evaluated 240 mg/day of the ginkgo biloba extract EGb 761. Retinal capillary blood flow increased significantly, by 0.44 mm/sec, in the ginkgo group ($P < 0.05$). Blood viscosity decreased at high, medium, and low shear rates (a measure of red blood cell strength). The results were –0.44, $P < 0.05$; –0.52, $P < 0.05$; and –2.88, $P < 0.01$, respectively. Oxygen transport efficiency increased significantly at all shear rates ($P < 0.05$). Erythrocyte rigidity decreased only at shear rates of 150 and 5 per second (–0.02 at both rates, $P < 0.05$). Erythrocyte MDA levels (a product of lipid peroxidation) also decreased (–0.92 × 10^{10} nmol/cell, $P < 0.05$), indicating that oxidative stress decreased. Overall, ginkgo use results in improved retinal capillary circulation without increasing blood glucose.

Summary

Ginkgo biloba is a very popular product that has been used for a variety of disease states. There are issues with the potential for bleeding and hemorrhage if combined with drugs or CAM supplements with antiplatelet effects. Doses of gingko biloba are variable: 120–240 mg/day for dementia, 120–160 mg/day for peripheral vascular disease, and 240 mg/day for retinopathy.[19] Gingko biloba is administered in divided doses, usually two or three times daily. Administration for 6–8 weeks is required to determine the benefit. Although ginkgo biloba may help in retinopathy, its role in lowering blood glucose and affecting insulin resistance in diabetes is unknown. Since ginkgo may affect insulin secretion, close monitoring of blood glucose and A1C is warranted.

FISH OIL (N-3 FATTY ACIDS)

N-3, or omega-3, fatty acids are another type of essential fatty acid (in addition to n-6, or GLA). There are two sources of n-3 fatty acids: plant oils and fish oils.[312] The plant oils contain ALA, and the main sources are walnut, flaxseed (linseed), canola, soybean, and olive. Fish oils are a source of n-3 long-chain polyunsaturated fatty acids. Certain fish, such as such as salmon, trout, halibut, mackerel, sturgeon, tuna, and sardines, are sources of n-3 fatty acids. The oils are high in the fatty acids eicosapentanoic acid and docosahexanoic acid.[312]

Fish oil is used for cardiovascular disease, specifically to treat high triglycerides, as well as for various inflammatory diseases, such as rheumatoid arthritis, psoriasis, inflammatory bowel disease, and dermatitis. Individuals have also used fish oil for a variety of other disorders, including asthma, renal disease, and psychiatric disorders.[19, 313] Interest in fish oil products for cardiovascular disease protection has stemmed from the observation that people with increased fish consumption had lower cardiovascular disease rates.[314] Since cardiovascular disease is the primary cause of mortality in diabetes, there is interest in use of fish oil possibly to diminish cardiovascular complications such as heart disease and stroke. There is also interest in use of fish oil in pre-diabetes because preliminary information indicates that fish oil consumption may reduce the risk of type 2 diabetes.[315] There are other reported uses, including hypertension treatment (in higher-than-recommended doses) and ischemic stroke prevention. Other potential benefits for which there is varying evidence include improvement of endothelial function, diminished oxidative stress, reduced albuminuria, and elevated C-reactive protein.[315]

Chemical Constituents and Mechanism of Action

The n-3 fatty acids are characterized by a structure that has several carbon atoms and several double bonds. It contains a double bond at the third carbon atom from the methyl end of the fatty acid chain, hence the name n-3 or omega-3.[314] The mechanism of action involves antithrombotic and anti-inflammatory effects due to competition with arachidonic acid in the cyclo-oxygenase and lipoxygenase pathways.[313] Thus, fish oil inhibits thromboxane A2, prostaglandin, and leukotriene production and enhances prostacyclin synthesis, thereby reducing platelet aggregation and promoting vasodilation. Fish oil also inhibits interleukin-1 and tumor necrosis factor-alpha production. Cardiac cell membrane stabilization is another potential property that may confer some antiarrhythmic effects.[312, 313] Other potential antiarrhythmic effects are related to maintenance of L-type calcium channels during cardiac stress and increased activity of cardiac microsomal calcium/magnesium-ATPase and inhibition of sodium channels.[312] Decreased secretion and increased clearance of very-low-density lipoproteins may help lower triglycerides.[313] There are many other theorized mechanisms of action, including altered metabolism of adhesion molecules such as vascular cell adhesion molecule-1, E-selectin, and intercellular adhesion molecule-1.[312]

Adverse Effects and Drug Interactions

Adverse effects of fish-oil intake include a "fishy after-taste" and belching, halitosis, heartburn, nausea, and loose stools.[19] Doses higher than 3 g/day may excessively inhibit platelet aggregation. Certain fish, such as shark, mackerel, and swordfish, may contain high levels of mercury, and fish from polluted waters may contain unacceptable levels of PCBs (polychlorinated biphenyls).[312, 313, 315] There is a dose-related effect on glucose, with doses higher than 3 g/day associated with increased blood glucose.[312, 315] There is also some concern that LDL concentrations may increase with higher doses, although the LDL particles may not be the atherogenic type.[312, 313, 315]

Additive effects may occur when taken with medications or other CAM supplements that have antiplatelet effects. However, consuming very high doses (>10 g/day) may actually increase risk of hemorrhagic stroke.[315] Oral contraceptives may interfere with the triglyceride-lowering effects of fish oils.[19]

Fish oil may have additive effects with antihypertensives, hypo-glycemics, and statins. Other effects include decreased hypertensive effects of cyclosporine and enhanced benefits with retinoids such as etretinate.[19]

Clinical Studies

Numerous studies have been published assessing use of fish oils for cardio-vascular disease and other illnesses. One of the largest studies prospectively evaluated fish oil supplementation as a secondary prevention in 11,324 individuals who had suffered a myocardial infarction.[288] In this multicenter, open-label study, GISSI, patients were randomized to daily doses of 1 g/day of n-3 fatty acid, 300 mg vitamin E, a combination of n-3 fatty acid and vitamin E, or placebo. After 3.5 years, the n-3 fatty acid group had a 10% reduction ($P = 0.048$) in the primary end point (death, nonfatal MI, or nonfatal stroke). Cardiovascular death was reduced by 17% (95% CI, 0.71–0.97), and all-cause mortality was reduced by 14% (95% CI, 0.76–0.97). There was no benefit seen in the vitamin E group. Although 15% of the subjects had diabetes, the researchers did not report the results in this group. Another study assessed the time to achieve benefit in the GISSI trial and found that risk of total mortality was significantly reduced after 3 months of treatment (RR = 0.59, or risk reduction of 41%, $P = 0.037$) and that after 4 months, risk of sudden death was significantly reduced (RR = 0.47, or risk reduction of 53%, $P = 0.048$).[316]

The Cochrane Collaboration published a review of 18 randomized, placebo-controlled trials assessing fish oil supplementation effects on death, lipids, and glucose control in patients with type 2 diabetes.[317] A total of 18 trials including 823 subjects were assessed. Study duration ranged from 2 to 24 weeks. A total of 14 trials reported triglyceride data, and overall this parameter was decreased by a mean of 0.56 mmol/l (~50 mg/dl) compared with placebo (95% CI, −0.71 to −0.40 mmol/l). Eleven trials reported LDL cholesterol data, and mean LDL was significantly increased by 9.2 mg/dl (0.24 mmol/l; $P = 0.01$) versus placebo. The evaluation noted that triglycerides were lowered to a greater extent in subjects with hypertriglyceridemia and that LDL increased the most in trials using higher doses and lasting longer than 2 months. There was no statistically significant effect on HDL cholesterol, fasting glucose, or A1C. However, the authors noted that there is a need for long-term studies that focus on cardiovascular end points assessing fish oil use in people with diabetes. There are two other analyses noting that fish oil use in diabetes decreases triglycerides by ~50 mg/dl (0.56 mmol/l) without adversely affecting A1C.[318, 319]

Summary

Fish oil has been widely used for cardiovascular protection. A systematic review has indicated that statins or fish oil are associated with decreased cardiac and overall mortality.[320] The ADA and AHA have recommended intake of two servings of fish per week.[312, 321] Other sources of n-3 fatty acids include fortified eggs and microalgae-derived oils. A recent report by the Agency for Health Care Research and Quality reviewed studies that assessed n-3 fatty acids in a variety of medical conditions, including diabetes.[322] The final report on the 18 studies in patients with diabetes indicated that the n-3 fatty acids lowered triglycerides compared with placebo, but did not affect total, HDL, or LDL cholesterol and did not affect fasting glucose or A1C. The report recommended that trials of n-3 fatty acids should assess baseline dietary consumption and that studies should quantify the source and specific n-3 acids in the supplement.

There is now a prescription product, Omacor, that contains 375 mg docosahexanoic acid and 465 mg eicosapentanoic acid.[323] It is approved for treating triglyceride concentrations higher than 500 mg/dl (5.65 mmol/l). At this time there is no proof that fish oil prevents development of type 2 diabetes, although its use may be of benefit in people with type 2 diabetes who have elevated triglycerides. Pregnant women should be cautioned regarding the consumption of fish because of the possibility of high mercury levels or PCBs. Commonly used doses of dietary supplements containing n-3 fatty acids for elevated triglycerides are from 1 g/day to 4 g/day.[19] At this time the best recommendation would be for patients to consume two to three servings a week of fish that are high in n-3 fatty acids.

POLICOSANOL (*Saccharum Officinarum* L.)

The most widely used policosanol product is extracted from sugar cane, *Saccharum officinarum*.[324] It is a mix of waxy substances consisting of alcohol components. One of the components, octosanol, is also obtained from other sources, such as wheat germ oil, alfalfa, or vegetable oil.[75] Policosanol has been widely used in Caribbean countries and South America to treat hyperlipidemia, including diabetes-related hyperlipidemia, as well as for intermittent claudication.

Chemical Constituents and Mechanism of Action

Policosanol is a high–molecular weight compound that contains a mix of eight primary aliphatic alcohols. Octacosanol comprises the largest part (>60%) of the mixture.[75, 324] Other important alcohols contained in the mixture include triacosanol and hexacosanol. Less important alcohols include tetracosanol, heptacosanol, nonacosanol, dotriacontanol, and tetratriacontanol.[19, 325]

The exact mechanism of lipid lowering is unknown, but hepatic cholesterol synthesis is inhibited and LDL degradation is enhanced.[19] LDL metabolism may also be improved by increased LDL binding, uptake, and breakdown in human fibroblasts.[325, 326] In intermittent claudication, policosanol affects the arachidonic acid cascade and decreases platelet aggregation.[19]

Adverse Effects and Drug Interactions

Relatively few side effects have been reported. They include erythema, dizziness, gastrointestinal upset, nasal and gum bleeding, insomnia, slight weight loss, and excessive urination.[19, 75] No adverse effects on weight, heart rate, blood pressure, or laboratory tests have been reported.[327] Additive effects may occur with antiplatelet agents, including prescription and nonprescription antiplatelet products, anti-inflammatories, Cox-2 inhibitors, and CAM supplements with antiplatelet effects.

Clinical Studies

One small randomized, double-blind, placebo-controlled study was done in 29 hyperlipidemic individuals with diet- or sulfonylurea-treated type 2 diabetes.[327] The patients had A1C <8% and fasting glucose <126 mg/dl (7.0 mmol/l) at randomization. After a 6-week lipid-lowering diet, subjects were randomized to policosanol (5 mg twice daily) or placebo for 12 weeks. Baseline LDL cholesterol decreased from 211 mg/dl (5.49 mmol/l) to 165 mg/dl (4.30 mmol/l) at end point in the poli-cosanol group ($P < 0.01$). In the placebo group, LDL cholesterol increased from 191 mg/dl (4.96 mmol/l) to 213 mg/dl (5.53 mmol/l; $P < 0.01$ for policosanol vs. placebo). Total cholesterol also decreased significantly in the policosanol group and was significantly lower than in the placebo group ($P < 0.01$ for both the decrease from baseline and versus placebo).

Another double-blind, randomized trial was done in 53 hyperlipidemic patients with type 2 diabetes.[328] Policosanol (10 mg daily) was compared with lovastatin (20 mg daily) for 12 weeks. Policosanol lowered LDL cholesterol by 20.4%, from a mean baseline of 205 mg/dl (5.33 mmol/l) to 161 mg/dl (4.18 mmol/l; $P < 0.001$), and lovastatin decreased LDL by 16.8%, from a mean baseline of 203 mg/dl (5.27 mmol/l) to 176 mg/dl (4.58 mmol/l; $P < 0.01$). Total cholesterol decreased significantly, by 14.2% and 14%, in the policosanol and lovastatin groups, respectively ($P < 0.0001$ in both groups). HDL cholesterol increased significantly, by 7.5% ($P < 0.01$), in the policosanol group but not in the lovastatin group. Triglycerides did not change in either group.

A meta-analysis of 29 randomized, double-blind, placebo-controlled studies found there was a significant lowering of LDL cholesterol in 1,528 patients on policosanol compared with 1,406 patients on placebo.[329] The weighted estimate of percentage change was a 23.7% decline in the policosanol group versus a 0.11% decrease in the placebo group ($P < 0.0001$ for policosanol vs. placebo).

One study that did not show benefit was a multicenter, randomized, double-blind, placebo-controlled trial in 143 German patients.[330] After a 6-week placebo run-in accompanied by dietary counseling, patients were randomized to placebo or one of four different strengths (10, 20, 40, or 80 mg daily every evening) of policosanol for 12 weeks. The primary end point was LDL cholesterol. Mean baseline LDL cholesterol decreased from 200 mg/dl (5.20 mmol/l) to 183 mg/dl (4.76 mmol/l) in the 10-mg group, from 185 mg/dl (4.80 mmol/l) to 175 mg/dl (4.55 mmol/l) in the 20-mg group, from 181 mg/dl (4.70 mmol/l) to 176 mg/dl (4.57 mmol/l) in the 40-mg group, and from 186 mg/dl (4.84 mmol/l) to 173 mg/dl (4.49 mmol/l) in the 80-mg group. The results were not significant for any of the policosanol groups or for placebo (decline from 181 mg/dl [4.70 mmol/l] to 166 mg/dl [4.31 mmol/l] in the placebo group). Secondary end points were also not significant (including triglycerides and total and HDL cholesterol). This trial excluded people with diabetes.

Summary

Several studies have evaluated policosanol use. One study in patients with type 2 diabetes showed a 17% decrease in LDL cholesterol after 12 weeks of policosanol (10 mg daily),[327] while another trial showed a 20.4% decrease.[328] In a 2-year trial, policosanol (10 mg/day) lowered baseline LDL from 206 mg/dl (5.35 mmol/l) to 155 mg/dl (4.02 mmol/l).[331] Policosanol has been used for up to 2 years for intermittent claudication, with improved treadmill walking distances.[332] Many of the studies have come from the same researchers in Cuba, using a Cuban product, and the results have generally been positive. Only a few studies have not shown benefit. One negative study used a wheat germ policosanol product.[333] Another study in German patients failed to find benefit from the same product that had been used in earlier studies.[330] In a comparison study, policosanol did not reduce total and LDL cholesterol as effectively as atorvastatin, a potent statin.[334] At this point, policosanol is a relatively benign product that may be of use when dosed at 10–20 mg/day for hyperlipidemia and 20 mg/day for intermittent claudication. However, people who are taking aspirin for risk reduction or are on antiplatelet agents should be warned about the possibility of bleeding interactions, although aspirin has been used in combination with policosanol.[325] Evidence regarding its effects on morbidity and mortality is missing. At this point statins have clearly shown benefit in cardiovascular outcomes, whereas policosanol has not; therefore, this product is not recommended for use.

GARLIC (*Allium sativum*)

Garlic, a member of the lily family, has been used in cooking for thousands of years.[19, 75] The name Allium is derived from the Celtic word *all* which means burning. Highly valued in ancient Egypt and ancient Chinese medicine, garlic has a rich history of thousands of years of medicinal use.[335] Garlic is a perennial plant with an odiferous bulb and a flowering stem that reaches 2–3 feet (about 1 meter) in height. The plant bears pinkish purplish flowers that bloom from midsummer to September. The medicinal activity is in the bulb.[75]

Garlic has been used for a variety of reasons, from warding off evil spirits to treating hyperlipidemia and hypertension, preventing cancer, and killing bacteria. Garlic has been reported to reduce blood glucose in animals and humans,[124, 140] but reviews of trials using garlic have not supported this.[336]

Chemical Constituents and Mechanism of Action

Garlic contains the sulfur-based chemical constituent alliin, which must be converted to the active form, allicin, by the enzyme alliinase. This reaction occurs when the garlic bulb is chewed or crushed.[75] The active constituents include allicin, ajoene, and other agents such as S-allyl-L-cysteine. Commercial garlic products may contain alliin, but not allicin or ajoene. Conversion requires alliinase, which is unstable in stomach acids. Dried garlic preparations may be effective only if the product is enteric coated to prevent gastric acid breakdown and permit release in the small intestine. Fresh garlic, however, is effective.[19, 75]

Allicin has antibacterial and antioxidant activity. Ajoene is formed by the acid-catalyzed reaction of two allicin molecules. It decreases the activity of factors needed for lipid synthesis by reducing the thiol group in coenzyme A and HMG-CoA reductase and by oxidizing NADPH. Ajoene has antiplatelet activity and interferes with thromboxane synthesis.[75] Animal research indicates that the constituents, S-methylcysteine sulfoxide and S-allylcysteine sulfoxide, may produce hypoglycemic effects.[19] Researchers have noted that garlic use may be associated with increased serum insulin and improved liver glycogen storage.[337]

Adverse Effects and Drug Interactions

Side effects of garlic include breath odor, mouth and gastrointestinal burning or irritation, heartburn, flatulence, allergic reactions, and, rarely, topical lesions and burns. There are case reports of spontaneous spinal epidural hematoma, retrobulbar hemorrhage, and postoperative bleeding associated with garlic use.[19, 75]

Bleeding may occur if a patient takes antiplatelet agents such as warfarin or aspirin or CAM supplements with antiplatelet activity such as ginkgo, ginger, feverfew, or others.[19] Garlic may induce CYP 3A4 isoenzyme activity, thus decreasing the effects of drugs that are metabolized through this pathway. Decreased efficacy of oral contraceptives, cyclosporine, protease inhibitors, calcium-channel blockers, certain statins, certain non-nucleoside reverse transcriptase inhibitors, certain anticonvulsants, certain macrolides, and other drugs may occur. Garlic oil may also inhibit CYP 2E1 activity and result in increased concentrations of ethanol, acetaminophen, and other products.[19]

Clinical Studies

A meta-analysis of garlic evaluated 13 randomized, double-blind, placebo-controlled trials that used garlic monopreparations, included subjects with total cholesterol >200 mg/dl (5.17 mmol/l), and evaluated total cholesterol as an end point.[338] The analysis found that garlic reduced total cholesterol more effectively than placebo ($P < 0.01$). The weighted mean difference was a decrease of 15.7 mg/dl (0.41 mmol/l; 95% CI, −25.6 to −5.7). The analysis also showed that for trials with better methodology there was no difference between garlic and placebo.

Another meta-analysis evaluated garlic use for cardiovascular risk factors.[336] At 8–12 weeks, studies that evaluated standardized garlic preparations showed decreases in total cholesterol of 19.2 mg/dl (0.50 mmol/l; 12 trials), decreases in LDL of 6.7 mg/dl (0.17 mmol/l; 10 trials), and decreases in triglycerides of 21.1 mg/dl (0.24 mmol/l; 13 trials). However, at 6 months the reductions were not maintained. HDL concentrations did not improve and decreased slightly. Another trial evaluated garlic in type 2 diabetes with newly diagnosed hyperlipidemia.[339] This was a single-blind, placebo-controlled study in 70 subjects. Total cholesterol decreased by 28 mg/dl (0.72 mmol/l; $P < 0.001$), LDL decreased by 30 mg/dl (0.78 mmol/l; $P < 0.001$), and HDL increased by 3.35 mg/dl (0.09 mmol/l; $P < 0.05$) in the garlic group. Triglycerides did not decrease. However, in this trial the patients were studied for only 12 weeks.

A meta-analysis of 8 trials evaluated the effect of garlic on mild hypertension.[340] Results indicated a modest decrease in systolic blood pressure (7.7 mmHg) and diastolic blood pressure (5 mmHg) compared with placebo. However, only three of the trials were conducted in hypertensive patients. Three of the trials showed a significant reduction in systolic pressure, and four showed a significant reduction in diastolic pressure.

The meta-analysis of garlic use for cardiovascular risk factors also evaluated effects on blood pressure in 23 trials.[336] Systolic blood pressure was significantly reduced in only one trial, and diastolic pressure was significantly reduced in three trials. Twelve trials evaluated blood glucose lowering. Only one showed a significant decrease, but it was in patients without diabetes. Therefore, the meta-analysis indicated a small, short-term benefit on lipids, an insignificant effect on blood pressure, and no significant decline in glucose in subjects with diabetes.

Summary

Garlic is commonly used for cardiovascular disease and other disease states related to diabetes. There are theoretical mechanisms for glucose reduction, but this has never been shown in humans. Recent work does however indicate that garlic may inhibit formation of advanced glycation end products, which are implicated in the etiology of diabetes-related microvascular complications.[341] Overall, garlic has shown only modest effects on hyperlipidemia. Therefore, patients should be told that garlic may be of benefit only in mild hyperlipidemia. Patients with diabetes generally need more aggressive lipid-lowering agents to insure that LDL cholesterol is <100 mg/dl (2.60 mmol/l) or, in some cases, <70 mg/dl (1.82 mmol/l). Effects on hypertension are also slight. People with diabetes may need more aggressive antihypertensive effects than garlic may provide. It is important that patients be instructed that antiplatelet activity is a serious potential problem, particularly if they are to have surgery or are on antiplatelet agents. For fresh garlic, the dose is 1 clove daily. Dried garlic powder preparations standardized to 1.3% allicin content have been used in studies. Dried garlic preparations should be enteric coated to prevent breakdown by stomach acids. In hyperlipidemia and hypertension studies, garlic extracts (600–1,200 mg/day in divided doses) have been used.[19]

GUGGUL (*Commiphora mukul*)

Guggul is also known as guggulipid or guggulu. It comes from the mukul myrrh tree, which is grown in India, and is the same genus as myrrh mentioned in the Bible. The plant is a thorny shrub or small tree that may grow to about 10 feet (3 meters) in height.[140] The bark of the tree exudes a gummy yellowish resin when injured, and this resin has been used in Ayurvedic medicine for thousands of years.[75, 342] Guggul has been used to treat acne, obesity, arthritis, and hyperlipidemia.

Chemical Constituents and Mechanism of Action

The proposed active constituents are the guggulsterone E and Z stereoisomers. One theorized mechanism is that guggul may decrease hepatic steroid production and increase LDL breakdown. Another theorized mechanism is that the guggulsterones may increase LDL cholesterol binding sites and increase LDL clearance. Increased cholesterol breakdown and excretion may also occur because the guggulsterones may act as antagonists at the farnesoid X receptor, the receptor that regulates conversion of cholesterol to bile acids. By acting as antagonists at the receptor, 7α-hydroxylase is released, stimulating cholesterol breakdown.[342] In obesity, guggul may stimulate thyroid activity and help increase metabolic rate.[75] It may also be of benefit in cardiac disease because it has fibrinolytic properties.

Adverse Effects and Drug Interactions

The most commonly reported adverse effects are gastrointestinal, including loose stools, diarrhea, and hiccups. Headache and rash have also been reported. Due to effects on platelets, bleeding reactions may occur. Guggul is thought to be an emmenagogue, which may cause spontaneous miscarriage; thus this product should not be used by pregnant women.[19]

The most significant drug interaction caution involves concomitant use of antiplatelet drugs or CAM supplements, due to the bleeding potential. Another significant drug interaction involves thyroid medications, since guggul may stimulate thyroid production. Hence, the dose of thyroid supplements may have to be adjusted. Guggul may also decrease bioavailability of propranolol and diltiazem.[75, 124] Preliminary information indicates that guggul may induce the CYP 3A4 isoenzyme system and thus decrease serum concentration of many medications, including some statins, calcium-channel blockers, certain angiotensin-receptor blockers, cyclosporine, and several others.[19]

Clinical Studies

Although there are several studies that have shown that guggul may reduce elevated lipids, there have often been problems with study design, including lack of randomization or a placebo control group. One trial with appropriate study design was a randomized, double-blind, placebo-controlled trial that evaluated 64 patients for 52 weeks.[343] The patients had a 12-week diet stabilization period, following a 4-week observation period. They then had 24 weeks of 50 mg twice daily guggul or placebo, followed by a 12-week washout. Total and LDL cholesterol and triglycerides declined significantly in the guggul group during treatment. Total cholesterol decreased by 25.2 mg/dl (0.65 mmol/l) from a baseline of 215.2 mg/dl (5.57 mmol/l; after diet), compared with a 7.6 mg/dl (0.20 mmol/l) increase in the placebo group from a baseline of 219.8 mg/dl (5.68 mmol/l; after diet) ($P < 0.01$ vs. placebo). LDL cholesterol decreased by 16.9 mg/dl (0.44 mmol/l) from a baseline of 135.1 mg/dl (3.51 mmol/l; after diet), and it increased by 4 mg/dl (0.10 mmol/l) in the placebo group from a baseline of 136.8 mg/dl (3.56 mmol/l) after diet) ($P < 0.01$ vs. placebo). Triglycerides decreased by 18 mg/dl (0.2 mmol/l) from baseline ($P < 0.05$) versus an increase of 5.5 mg/dl (0.06 mmol/l) in the placebo group. Lipids then increased at the end of the washout period.

A more recent study indicates that guggul may not be as effective as previously thought. In this randomized, double-blind, placebo-controlled trial evaluating 103 subjects with hyperlipidemia,[344] the subjects were randomized to placebo or two different standardized doses of guggul containing 2.5% guggulsterones: 1,000 mg three times daily (75 mg guggulsterones/day) or 2,000 mg three times daily (150 mg guggulsterones/day). The mean baseline LDL values were 160 mg/dl (4.16 mmol/l), 156 mg/dl (4.06 mmol/l), and 161 mg/dl (4.19 mmol/l) in the placebo, 75-mg, and 150-mg guggulsterone/day groups, respectively.

After 8 weeks, the placebo group had a 5% decrease in LDL cholesterol, whereas LDL increased by 4% and 5% in the lower- and higher-dose guggul groups, respectively ($P = 0.01$ and $P = 0.06$ vs. placebo, respectively). HDL cholesterol decreased in both guggul groups and increased slightly in the placebo group. In subjects with LDL >160 mg/dl (4.16 mmol/l), triglycerides decreased significantly, by 14% and 10% in the lower- and higher-dose groups, respectively ($P = 0.02$ and $P = 0.03$ vs. placebo, respectively). The increased LDL results are consistent with a recent case report of an individual who also experienced an increase in LDL cholesterol instead of a decrease.[345]

Summary

Guggul is an Ayurvedic plant product that has increased in popularity in the U.S. It is a resin that is reported to decrease total and LDL cholesterol. Most of the favorable studies have been conducted in India. However, a recent study with good design conducted in the U.S. indicated that total and LDL cholesterol may actually increase.[344] Guggul may produce adverse gastrointestinal effects, enhance the effects of thyroid supplements, and possibly decrease the effects of many medications that patients with diabetes may be taking, including certain statins. There is potential for bleeding reactions, especially if combined with antiplatelet agents. Supplements containing guggul should not be taken by pregnant women. The dose used for hyperlipidemia is 75–150 mg daily of standardized guggulsterones. There is conflicting evidence regarding benefit of guggul, and its use is not advocated.

RED YEAST RICE (*Monascus purpureus* Went)

Red yeast rice is also known as red yeast or XueZhiKang. The *Monascus purpureus* yeast, made through a fermentation process using rice,[19, 75] contains monacolin K, or lovastatin, as well as other HMG-CoA reductase inhibitory products. The ancient Chinese pharmacopeia describes red yeast. It has been used to make rice wine and is used as a food preservative and coloring agent for meat and fish. It is also used as a medicinal food to promote "blood circulation" and to treat hyperlipidemia.[346]

Chemical Constituents and Mechanism of Action

The product contains several monacolins, including lovastatin and hydroxy acids.[75] It has HMG-CoA reductase inhibitory activity to prevent cholesterol formation. Other active ingredients include beta-sitosterol, stigmasterol, campesterol, isoflavones, and saponins.[19, 124] Another product, citrinin, may be inadvertently produced by the yeast and is a nephrotoxic agent.[19, 75]

Adverse Effects and Drug Interactions

Many consider red yeast rice to be another statin, and it may have the same side effects as other statins. Red yeast rice may cause gastrointestinal upset and increased liver function tests as well as allergic reactions. It may also cause myalgias and has the potential to cause rhabdomyolysis. If the product inadvertently contains citrinin, nephrotoxicity may occur.[19, 75]

Because of the lipid-lowering effects, there may be additive cholesterol lowering with other antihyperlipidemic agents. Grapefruit may increase serum concentrations, since lovastatin is metabolized through CYP 3A4 and grapefruit is a CYP 3A4 inhibitor.[19] Other medications with similar CYP 3A4 inhibition may produce the same increased serum concentrations, such as certain macrolides, azole antifungals, protease inhibitors, and the antidepressant nefazodone. On the other hand, St. John's wort, phenobarbital, carbamazepine, and phenytoin may reduce serum concentrations because they induce CYP 3A4 isoenzymes. In combination with gemfibrozil there is a theoretical concern about rhabdomyolysis. With high-dose niacin there is also the theoretical potential for myopathy and liver toxicity. Concomitant use with thyroid supplements may result in thyroid function abnormalities.[19] Red yeast rice use may result in lower CoQ10 serum concentrations.

Clinical Studies

A randomized, double-blind, placebo-controlled trial evaluated use of a proprietary Chinese supplement in 83 patients with hyperlipidemia.[347] Patients took placebo or 2.4 g/day of the product for 12 weeks. Mean baseline cholesterol decreased from 254 mg/dl (6.57 mmol/l) to 210 mg/dl (5.43 mmol/l) in the red yeast rice group at 12 weeks ($P < 0.05$ vs. baseline), and in the placebo group baseline cholesterol decreased from 255 mg/dl (6.59 mmol/l) to only 250 mg/dl (6.47 mmol/l). LDL cholesterol decreased from 173 mg/dl (4.47 mmol/l) at baseline to 135 mg/dl (3.49 mmol/l) at 12 weeks in the red yeast rice group ($P < 0.001$). The LDL decrease was from 180 mg/dl (4.65 mmol/l) at baseline to 175 mg/dl (4.53 mmol/l) in the placebo group ($P < 0.001$ for red yeast rice at 12 weeks vs. placebo). Triglycerides also decreased in the red yeast rice group and were 124 mg/dl (1.4 mmol/l) versus 146 mg/dl (1.65 mmol/l) in the placebo group ($P = 0.05$ for red yeast rice vs. placebo). There were no changes in HDL cholesterol in either group.

Summary

Use of the product called Cholestin as a dietary supplement was controversial because it contained a specific monacolin thought to be lovastatin. The FDA ruled that the manufacturer should remove this ingredient, since it was similar to the prescription drug. Therefore, although red yeast rice is still available as a dietary supplement, it is not in the product Cholestin. A typical dose is 1,200 mg twice daily with food. This dose contains ~9.6 mg statins, 7.2 mg as lovastatin.[347] This product has not been evaluated in patients with diabetes, and the potential for interactions with statins and many other medications makes this a product that should not be recommended.

ST. JOHN'S WORT (*Hypericum perforatum* L.)

St. John's wort is a perennial that grows throughout the U.S., Canada, and Europe. The plant has a rich history. There are many species in the genus *Hypericum*, a name that came from the Greek words *hyper* and *eikon* meaning "over an apparition," since the plant was used to fend off evil spirits. The word *perforatum* is used because the translucent leaf glands resemble perforations. St. John's wort may grow up to about 5 feet (1.5 meters) in height. Its bright flowers bloom in late June (on the feast day of St. John), and the flowering top is used in various commercial products.[75] It has been used for a variety of reasons including antiviral and antibacterial effects. However, it is primarily used to treat depression, anxiety, and insomnia. Because many people with diabetes have depression, a discussion of St. John's wort is warranted.

Chemical Constituents and Mechanism of Action

St. John's wort contains the chemical constituents naphthodianthrones, flavonoids, phloroglucinols (including hyperforin), and essential oils. The naphthodianthrones include hypericin and hypericin-like substances (pseudohypericin, isohypericin, protohypericin). The flavonoids include hyperin, rutin, quercetin, and biflavones.[75]

Early in vitro research led many researchers to think that MAO inhibition was the mechanism of St. John's wort's antidepressant effects. However, recent studies have indicated that MAO inhibition does occur but only with high concentrations of the hypericum constituents, not those found in commercial extracts.[348]

The main ingredients thought to be responsible for the antidepressant activity are hypericin and hyperforin. Some researchers think the constituent most likely to result in antidepressant effects is hyperforin,[24] but many trials have used the hypericin extract. The mechanism is now thought to be inhibition of reuptake of serotonin, norepinephrine, and dopamine.[349] Other neurotransmitters that are also affected include gamma-aminobutyric acid and glutamate.[350]

Adverse Effects and Drug Interactions

Side effects of St. John's wort include phototoxicity,[351] as well as sleep difficulties, gastrointestinal upset, anxiety, and withdrawal-like symptoms when discontinued abruptly.[352] Photosensitivity may occur. St. John's wort may also increase thyroid-stimulating hormone.[353, 354] Overall, a systematic review indicated that St. John's wort is well tolerated, and adverse effects in postmarketing surveillance studies evaluating 34,804 patients have ranged from 0% to 6%.[355] Four large surveillance studies included 14,245 subjects and calculated a rate of adverse effects ranging from 0.1% to 2.4% and a drop-out rate of 0.1–0.9% secondary to adverse effects.[355]

St. John's wort has been found to produce serotonin syndrome when combined with serotonergic agents such as fluoxetine (Prozac).[356] Other serotonergic drugs include sertraline (Zoloft) and paroxetine (Paxil). Through different effects on P-glycoprotein modulation and CYP 3A4 and 2C9 isoenzyme system induction, St. John's wort may decrease serum concentrations of several drugs that a patient with diabetes may be taking.[19, 350] These drugs include digoxin, oral contraceptives, cyclosporine, warfarin, angiotensin-receptor blockers, theophylline, certain statins, and protease inhibitors.[357] Additive sedation may also occur when combined with narcotics.[19]

Clinical Studies

St. John's wort has been compared with placebo and traditional antidepressants. A Cochrane review assessed 27 randomized, controlled studies (involving 2,291 patients) comparing St. John's wort to placebo or other antidepressants.[358] Follow-up ranged from 12 to 26 weeks. In 14 studies, more patients responded to St. John's wort than to placebo ($P < 0.001$). Relative benefit increase was 140% (95% CI, 70–239). In five studies there was no difference in response between St. John's wort and low-dose antidepressants. Fewer side effects were reported with St. John's wort than with antidepressants (28% vs. 45%, $P = 0.002$).

Another study reported greater efficacy of St. John's wort than placebo but equal efficacy when compared with the tricyclic antidepressant imipramine.[359] St. John's wort has been found equal in efficacy to the antidepressants fluoxetine[360] and sertraline.[361] A recent study, however, reported no benefits for major depression.[362] Numerous studies continue to be published; some confirm the efficacy of St. John's wort in mild-to-moderate depression. Other trials do not corroborate this effect, particularly for severe depression.[363] However, in a trial evaluating patients with severe depression, there was no difference between the St. John's wort group and the comparator groups on sertraline or placebo.[363] Two more recent trials have shown that St. John's wort is as effective as paroxetine[364] and more effective than fluoxetine.[365]

Summary

St. John's wort is one of the most highly used CAM supplements and has been found to be useful for mild-to-moderate depression. Many people with diabetes are depressed, and these patients may be tempted to use "natural" products to treat their mood disorder. St. John's wort has been found to be more effective than placebo and in many cases as effective as traditional antidepressants. As with standard antidepressants, it may take several weeks to see a therapeutic benefit. Doses of St. John's wort are 300–600 mg three times daily. Standardized extracts used in studies include 0.3% hypericin and the hyperforin-stabilized version of this extract.

If a clinician finds that a patient is taking St. John's wort and wants to be respectful of that decision, several counseling points are important. Patients should be counseled to wear sunscreen and sunglasses when using St. John's wort and to gradually taper the dosage when discontinuing this product. Patients should be encouraged to inform their health care providers if they are taking St. John's wort, particularly because of the potential for drug interactions with medications that diabetes patients might be using, such as certain statins, certain antihypertensives, cyclosporine, digoxin, warfarin, and other important medications. Patients should be told that abrupt discontinuation of St. John's wort could result in dangerously increased serum concentrations of drugs that normally have decreased concentrations during coadministration. Also, if St. John's wort is added to some of these same drugs, serum concentrations of these drugs may fall below therapeutic levels.

Because of overall safety and efficacy concerns and the possibility of drug interactions, the use of St. John's wort is not advocated. If depression is suspected, the patient should be thoroughly evaluated to rule out other causes, such as hypothyroidism or other disease states. The use of a conventional antidepressant should be encouraged rather than allowing the patient to start or discontinue the use of a CAM supplement at will. Depression is a serious illness that may be successfully treated with conventional medications and/or behavioral therapies.

Table 3. Botanical and Nonbotanical CAM Supplements that May Treat Complications of Diabetes

Product	Chemical Constituents	Mechanism of Action	Side Effects & Drug Interactions
Alpha-Lipoic Acid (ALA)	Disulfide compound synthesized in the liver [266–268]	• ↑ insulin sensitivity • Functions as antioxidant to: - scavenge free radicals - regenerate endogenous antioxidants (vitamins C and E, glutathione) - metal chelating activity - stimulates glucose transporter systems and ↑ glucose transport - may help protect against impaired insulin-stimulated protein kinase-B activation. [267–271]	*Side effects:* • Nausea, vomiting, vertigo [268] • Possible skin allergies [19,268] • ↓ triiodothyronine levels [19] *Drug interactions:* • Possible hypoglycemia if combined with secretagogues [268] • Mineral deficiency • Toxicity in thiamine deficiency • May be bound by antacids [19]

| Vitamin E | • Fat-soluble vitamin consisting of 8 stereoisomers [19,279] | • Antioxidant activity to prevent free radical formation
• Anti-inflammatory effects to possibly ↓ atherosclerosis
• May serve as a protective antioxidant in renal failure [19,279,280] | *Side effects:*
• GI upset, headache, blurred vision, rash [19]
• Heart failure [281]
• Higher doses associated with ↑ mortality [282]
• Bleeding reactions with high doses [279,283]
Drug interactions:
• Bleeding reactions if high doses combined with antiplatelets [19,283]
• ↓ beneficial effect of statins on HDL [284]
• ↓ vitamin K effects with high vitamin E doses [19]
• Orlistat, bile acid sequestrants, mineral oil bind vitamin E [19]
• Phenytoin, phenobarbital, carbamazepine ↓ vitamin E levels [19] |

(Continued)

Table 3. (*Continued*)

Product	Chemical Constituents	Mechanism of Action	Side Effects & Drug Interactions
Gamma-Linolenic Acid (GLA)	Omega-6 essential fatty acid [19,75]	GLA is converted to dihomo-gamma-linolenic acid and arachidonic acid, prostaglandin precursors that • Regulate platelet aggregation • Maintain blood flow in small blood vessels [19,75,295]	*Side effects:* • Headache, GI upset • Case reports of bleeding-time prolongation • Case report of seizures [19,75] *Drug interactions:* • Theoretical interaction with phenothiazines with resulting seizure activity [19,75]

Ginkgo Biloba	• Flavonoids (ginkgo-flavone glycosides) • Terpenoids - ginkgolides - bilobalides [19,75,300]	• Flavone glycosides have antioxidant activity and inhibit platelet aggregation • Ginkgolides may improve circulation and inhibit platelet activating factor • Bilobalides thought to be neuroprotective • May affect insulin secretion [19,75,300]	*Side effects:* • Headache • GI upset • Bleeding reactions • Seizures if handling or eating the seeds [19,75,302] *Drug interactions:* • Bleeding reactions if combined with drugs or CAM supplements having antiplatelet properties [302] • May slightly ↑ serum concentrations of certain drugs including some antipsychotics, cardiac medications, warfarin, caffeine, and some sulfonylureas; effects thought to be variable [19,75] • Coma when combined with trazodone [303] • ↓ alprazolam concentrations 17% [304]

(Continued)

Table 3. (*Continued*)

Product	Chemical Constituents	Mechanism of Action	Side Effects & Drug Interactions
Fish Oil	• n-3 fatty acids [314]	• Antithrombotic effects [313] • Anti-inflammatory effects due to arachidonic acid cascade inhibition [313] • Inhibits interleukin-1 and tumor necrosis factor-alpha [312,313] • ↓ secretion and ↑ clearance of VLDLs [313] • Altered metabolism of adhesion molecules [313] - vascular cell adhesion molecule-1 - e-selectin - intercellular adhesion molecule-1	*Side effects:* • Fishy after-taste • GI upset • Halitosis [19] • ↑ mercury or polychlorinated biphenyls [312,313] • Doses >3 g/day may result in ↑ glucose [312,315] • High doses may ↑ nonatherogenic LDL particles [312,313,315] *Drug interactions:* • Additive bleeding if high doses taken with antiplatelet agents [315] • Possible hypoglycemia if combined with secretagogues [19]

| Policosanol | • Composed of 8 primary aliphatic alcohols, including
- octacosanol
- triacosanol
- hexacosanol
- others
[75,324] | • Inhibits hepatic cholesterol synthesis
• Enhanced LDL breakdown
• ↓ platelet aggregation [75,324,325,326] | • Possible additive effects with antihypertensives or statins [19]
• ↓ hypertensive effects of cyclosporine [19]
• ↑ benefits with retinoids [19]

Side effects:
• Erythema
• Dizziness
• GI upset
• Mucosal tissue bleeding [19,75]

Drug interactions:
• Possible additive bleeding with antiplatelet medications and CAM supplements [19,75] |

(Continued)

Table 3. (*Continued*)

Product	Chemical Constituents	Mechanism of Action	Side Effects & Drug Interactions
Garlic	• Alliin; must be converted to allicin (active form) by the enzyme allinase • Ajoene; formed by acid-catalyzed reaction from 2 allicin molecules • Allylpropyl disulfide [19,75]	• Antioxidant activity • Allicin may ↑ levels of catylase and glutathione peroxidase activity • Ajoene ↓ the activity of factors needed for lipid synthesis by reducing the thiol group in coenzyme A and HMG-CoA reductase and by oxidizing NADPH • Ajoene has antiplatelet activity and interferes with thromboxane synthesis and ↓ platelet activity • Allopropyl disulfide may ↓ blood glucose and ↑ insulin • ↑ serum insulin and improved hepatic glycogen storage [19,75,337]	*Side effects:* • ↑ gastrointestinal upset • Bleeding reactions [19,75] *Drug interactions:* • Additive antiplatelet effects when combined with drugs or CAM supplements having antiplatelet properties [19,75] • May induce CYP450 3A4, thus ↓ effects of many drugs (oral contraceptives, cyclosporine, calcium-channel blockers, certain statins, certain anticonvulsants, certain macrolides) [19] • May inhibit CYP450 2E1, thus may ↑ concentrations of ethanol, acetaminophen, and other drugs [19]

| Guggul | • Guggulsterone E and Z stereoisomers [342] | • May ↓ hepatic cholesterol synthesis [342]
• ↑ LDL cholesterol binding sites and ↑ LDL clearance [342]
• Antagonist at farnesoid X receptor so stimulates cholesterol breakdown [342]
• May stimulate thyroid activity [75,140] | *Side effects:*
• GI upset
• Hiccups
• Headache
• Rash
• Spontaneous miscarriage [19,342]

Drug interactions:
• Possible additive bleeding if used with antiplatelet medications or CAM supplements [19,342]
• Additive effects with thyroid supplements [75,140]
• ↓ bioavailability of propranolol and diltiazem [75,124]
• Possible CYP450 3A4 inducer; may ↓ serum concentrations of many drugs (calcium channel blockers, steroids, estrogens, etc.) [19] |

(Continued)

Table 3. (*Continued*)

Product	Chemical Constituents	Mechanism of Action	Side Effects & Drug Interactions

Red Yeast Rice	• Monacolin K
	• Hydroxy acids
	• Other ingredients
	  - beta sitosterol
	  - stigmasterol
	  - campesterol
	  - isoflavones
	  - saponins
	[19,124]
		• HMG-CoA reductase inhibition [19,346,347]	*Side effects:*
			• GI upset [19]
			• ↑ liver function enzymes [19]
			• Myalgias [19]
			• Allergies [19]
			• Citrinin may cause nephrotoxicity [19,75]
			Drug interactions:
			• Possible increased effects with CYP450 3A4 inhibitors (macrolides, azole antifungals, nefazodone, protease inhibitors) [19]
			• Possible rhabdomyolysis if used with gemfibrozil or niacin [19]
			• Thyroid function abnormalities if combined with thyroid supplements [19]
			• May ↓ CoQ10 concentrations [19]

| St. John's wort | • Hypericin
• Hyperforin
[19,24,75] | • Serotonergic activity as well as possible effects on other neurotransmitters [19,24,75,349,350] | *Side effects:*
• Phototoxicity
• Gastrointestinal upset, anxiety
• ↑ thyroid-stimulating hormone
• Withdrawal symptoms when discontinued abruptly [19,75,350,352,353,354]
Drug interactions:
• Induces metabolism of certain drugs, thereby decreasing their serum concentrations (certain antihypertensives, certain statins, warfarin, digoxin, oral contraceptives, cyclosporine, protease inhibitors) [350,357]
• Serotonin syndrome if combined with serotonergic drugs such as paroxetine or fluoxetine [19,356] |

5.

Other CAM Products

There are hundreds of CAM supplements that people may use for diabetes and related comorbidities.[366] Yeh, et al, have completed a systematic review of herbs and dietary supplements for glycemic control.[366] That comprehensive review discussed many of the supplements covered in this book, but also included other products, such as *Bauhinia forficata*, *Myrcia uniflora*, and certain combination products. The reader may find it a valuable resource. The quality of evidence for products reviewed was assessed using the U.S. Preventive Services Task Force criteria[367] and the American Diabetes Association evidence-grading system[368] for clinical practice recommendations.

Many other products are emerging in importance because of their ability to diminish insulin resistance or improve cardiovascular health. L-carnitine is one example. Synthesized from lysine and methionine, L-β-hydroxy-γ-N-trimethylaminobutyric acid, or L-carnitine, has a role in lipid metabolism and is a cofactor for mitochondrial β-oxidation of fatty acids. It helps transport acetyl groups across the mitochondrial membrane and also assists in glucose transport.[369] Although it has been used as a weight-loss supplement with little supporting evidence, studies in small numbers of patients using intravenous L-carnitine have shown improvement in glucose disposal.[370] Used orally, it has been shown to decrease fasting glucose, but with a concomitant increase in triglycerides.[371] L-carnitine has also been evaluated for peripheral neuropathy with some success.[372,373]

Another example of a product of emerging interest is dark chocolate. There has been interest in its medicinal properties because of epidemiological studies in Kuna Indians, who live off the coast of Panama and have a very low occurrence of cardiovascular disease (hypertension, dyslipidemia) and diabetes.[374] A theorized explanation is the high consumption of cocoa-rich beverages. Because of the polyphenol content of (−)-epicatechin and (+)-catechin and procyanidins (the oligomers of epicatechin and/or catechin), chocolate may regulate nitric oxide. The flavanols may increase nitric oxide bioavailability and thus enhance insulin sensitivity, produce vessel relaxation, and decrease blood pressure.[374] Dark chocolate has been shown to decrease fasting glucose and insulin concentrations as well as glucose response to OGTT.[374] In people with hypertension, dark chocolate has also been shown to decrease blood pressure and LDL cholesterol and to improve insulin sensitivity.[375] Foods that are high in flavanols, such as certain fruits; berries; wine; green, oolong, or black tea; and dark chocolate may have antioxidant effects and attenuate LDL oxidation. Interestingly, the cocoa powder and extracts have greater antioxidant capacity than green or black tea, red wine, berries, or garlic.[376] The mechanism of antioxidant effects is thought to consist of trapping free radicals and chelating redox-active metals because of the presence of a catechol group in one of the rings of the structure.[376] However, it is important that clinicians stress to their patients that information is emerging and benefit is shown only with dark chocolate containing flavanols, not with confectionery chocolate, which has very low flavanol content.

Many patients are often hopeful and are looking for answers, new cures, and possible uses of new popular supplements. They will often embrace products before there is adequate research. An example is that of hoodia (*Hoodia gordonii* Masson, Sweet ex Decne, Asclepiadaceae). This succulent cactus-like African plant has become a very popular weight-loss supplement.[19] Hoodia is now part of a million dollar industry in the U.S., in spite of the fact that there are no published clinical trials to support the appetite-suppressant effects. Contributing to the problem of lack of regulation is that many products supposedly containing hoodia have been discovered actually not to contain the plant.[377]

In spite of enthusiasm for new clinical findings, the clinician is directed to the statement by the ADA on unproven therapies, which acknowledges the widespread use of alternative therapies and the need for cautious evaluation of these products.[378]

6.

Closing Comments and Advice for Clinicians

Because of the increasing popularity of CAM, clinicians may find themselves serving as a resource for diabetes patients who are interested in using such therapies. Clinicians should therefore strive to familiarize themselves with current research in this area. An open-minded, yet evidence-based approach is important. Many patients may be reluctant to inform their health care providers of CAM supplement use, and an open mind is critical to ensuring the patient is not alienated. If a clinician is well-informed regarding the different types of CAM supplements, then a patient may be more likely to discuss his or her interest in using these products.

Patients with diabetes who are considering use of CAM supplements are likely to be actively involved in their own health care and should be congratulated for their efforts. Clinicians should strive to encourage open communication about CAM supplement use and to provide information on efficacy as well as potential adverse effects and drug interactions. A discussion of regulation and manufacturing issues is also important, and it is essential to discourage the use of dangerous or ineffective products or those for which there is little evidence.

Patients should be asked at each visit whether they have started or stopped taking any CAM supplements. It is vital to keep educating the patient that CAM supplements are not benign and that their use may result in adverse effects and interactions with comorbid diseases, drugs, nutrients, or even other CAM supplements. Clinicians should know the entire spectrum of products the patient is using to provide the best possible care. Patients should be educated regarding the possibility of adverse effects during or after surgery, and clinicians should educate their patients to discontinue CAM supplements 1–2 weeks before surgery.

Advise patients that if supplements are used, they should be used in addition to the essential elements of the diabetes care regimen, such as medications, meal planning, and physical activity. It is especially important to stress that CAM supplements should not replace prescribed medications.

Inform patients that even though they may regard CAM supplements as being natural, the supplements are not necessarily safer than other products. Because most of the products are not subject to rigorous government safety and efficacy testing, they may even be more dangerous than conventional medications.

Patients should be encouraged to do research on a product before they begin taking it, particularly since many products are very expensive and may provide questionable health benefits. There is less published evidence for use of CAM supplements than for conventional diabetes medications. There is insufficient information to support universal use of these products by patients with diabetes, and again the clinician is referred to the American Diabetes Association's statement on unproven therapies.[378]

Teach patients to read labels carefully, and to look for telephone numbers, addresses, and websites on the labels of products. Patients should be encouraged to ask questions of the manufacturers. If a manufacturer is readily willing to supply published information rather than patient testimonials, that may be an indicator of a more reliable company.

Educate patients that it is best to compare ingredients when doing repeat purchasing to make sure that amounts, ingredients, and doses do not vary. Patients should be cautioned not to change brands continually. It is especially important that patients be taught to be wary of buying several different products that may duplicate the same ingredient and possibly inadvertently result in toxicity. Advise patients that they may wish to save a few pills in the bottle should the need arise to perform an assay of the product (in case of adverse effects).

Encourage patients to purchase products that are standardized whenever possible. Encourage patients to buy products from companies that invest in research and meet good manufacturing practice guidelines, as noted on the product label, to ensure product purity and safety. Recent problems have included contamination of products with ingredients that were not listed on the label. Tell patients that if possible they should buy products that have been evaluated through the Dietary Supplement Verification Program by the U.S. Pharmacopeia or NSF International or that come from companies involved in National Institutes of Health or other reliably sponsored research.

Tell patients about the FDA website that provides information for supplement users, "Tips for the Savvy Supplement User" (http://www.cfsan.fda.gov/~dms/ds-savvy.html). For older individuals, the clinician may suggest "Tips for Older Dietary Supplement Users" (http://www.cfsan.fda.gov/~dms/ds-savv2.html). Certain individuals, such as elderly people, pregnant or lactating women, and children warrant special caution, and CAM supplement use should be discouraged.

Inform patients that if they wish to try CAM supplements, they should consider single-ingredient rather than multiple-ingredient products. If an adverse effect or a worsening blood glucose level or other important clinical end point occurs, it will be easier to determine which substance may be responsible.

Patients should consider starting with a small dose of a product and working up to the recommended dose to determine whether the supplement has any effect on blood glucose levels and to avoid dose-related adverse effects. For some products it may take several weeks to determine whether there is an adequate effect on blood glucose. Ask patients to consider using the product for only a limited time to evaluate the effect. If there is no benefit, then discontinue use of the product.

Advise patients to monitor their blood glucose levels frequently when taking any type of CAM supplements and to share any concerns about changes in blood glucose with their health care team. Remind patients that using CAM supplements will not undo damage caused by an unhealthy lifestyle or unhealthy behaviors.

Advise patients to keep records to assess progress toward desired effects such as improvements in blood glucose, lipid profile, blood pressure, weight, neuropathy symptoms, and other aspects of diabetes care.

One of the most significant roles of a clinician is to help patients identify what they hope to achieve when using CAM supplements and to encourage them to keep records of the beneficial and adverse effects and to evaluate the impact on diabetes care. It is also important for clinicians to ask patients if they have stopped CAM supplement use. In the past, many clinicians may have been reluctant to establish a dialogue about their patients' attitudes toward CAM supplements because of a lack of confidence in their own knowledge of these products. Perhaps this book can help alleviate these concerns and will enhance the clinician-patient relationship. However, it remains imperative to emphasize that none of the CAM supplements discussed in this book have demonstrated achievement of American Diabetes Association–recommended goals for A1C, blood pressure, or lipids.

CASE STUDY

A postmenopausal woman with diabetes who has retinopathy and peripheral neuropathy asks her clinician about using CAM supplements to treat her diabetes and complications of diabetes. In addition to diabetes, she has hypertension, hyperlipidemia, intermittent claudication, and depression. She is taking Metaglip (a combination of metformin plus glyburide), Crestor (rosuvastatin, to treat hyperlipidemia), Cozaar (an angiotensin-receptor blocker to treat hypertension), Prempro (conjugated estrogens plus medroxyprogesterone acetate for hormone replacement therapy), and Zoloft (sertraline, a serotonin-specific reuptake inhibitor

[SSRI] antidepressant). The patient asks about cinnamon, gymnema, fenugreek, bitter melon, and ginseng to supplement her sulfonylurea-metformin treatment.

Questions for Discussion

1. Can these help her diabetes?
2. What CAM supplements may be useful for the diabetes-related complications?
3. What potential drug interactions may occur if the patient uses CAM supplements?

Discussion

Like many of the products discussed in the book, the CAM supplements the patient is asking about have been used to treat diabetes. Although cinnamon or bitter melon could be consumed as foods, potential drug interactions may occur with use of the other CAM supplements. For example, additive hypoglycemia may occur with the sulfonylurea-metformin combination and these agents.

Agents that may be useful for peripheral neuropathy are alpha-lipoic acid and gamma-linolenic acid. For the retinopathy, pine bark extract and bilberry may be considered. Other supplements that may be of some benefit in treating her other conditions are garlic for hypertension and hyperlipidemia, gingko for the intermittent claudication, and St. John's wort for depression.

Her clinician should educate her about the following cautions: Ginseng may attenuate the beneficial effects of her antihypertensive medication and may produce additive estrogenic effects with her hormone replacement therapy. St. John's wort may produce serotonin syndrome in combination with the SSRI. Finally, St. John's wort may lower blood levels of her antihypertensive medication, and she may experience an increase in blood pressure. If St. John's wort is used and then stopped, the dose of the antihypertensive may have to be adjusted. Specifically, the dose of the antihypertensive may have to be increased if St. John's wort is taken and then decreased if St. John's wort is stopped.

Any of the agents she decides to try should be standardized extracts from a reputable manufacturer, and they should be tried one at a time to determine the effect on her diabetes and comorbidities.

References

1. Centers for Disease Control: National Diabetes Fact Sheet. Available at http://www.cdc.gov/diabetes/pubs/factsheet05.htm. Accessed February 28, 2006.

2. Annual industry overview. *Nutr Bus J* 2002;May/Jun.

3. What is Complementary and Alternative Medicine? Available at http://nccam.nih.gov/health/whatiscam. Accessed May 21, 2006.

4. U.S. Food and Drug Administration Center for Food Safety and Applied Nutrition: Dietary Supplement Health and Education Act of 1994. Available at http://www.cfsan.fda.gov/~dms/dietsupp.html. Accessed May 21, 2006.

5. Overview of dietary supplements. Available at http://www.cfsan.fda.gov/~dms/ds-oview.html. Accessed May 21, 2006.

6. Eisenberg DM, Kessler RC, Foster C, Norlock FE, Calkins DR, Delbanco TL: Unconventional medicine in the United States: prevalence, costs, and patterns of use. *N Engl J Med* 1993;328:246–252.

7. Day C: Are herbal remedies of use in diabetes? *Diabetic Med* 2005;22 (Suppl. 1):10–12.

8. Bailey CJ, Day C: Traditional plant medicines as treatments for diabetes. *Diabetes Care* 1989;12:553–564.

9. Bailey CJ, Day C: Metformin: its botanical background. *Pract Diab Int* 2004;21:115–17.

10. Egede LE, Ye X, Zeng D, Silverstein MD: The prevalence and pattern of complementary and alternative medicine use in individuals with diabetes. *Diabetes Care* 2002;25:324–329.

11. Wolsko PM, Solondz DK, Phillips RS, et al.: Lack of herbal supplement characterization in published randomized controlled trials. *Am J Med* 2005;118:1087–1093.

12. Eisenberg DM, Davis RB, Ettner SL, et al.: Trends in alternative medicine use in the United States, 1990–1997: results of a follow-up national survey. *JAMA* 1998;280:1569–1575.

13. Shaw D, Leon C, Koley S, Murray V: Traditional remedies and food supplements: a 5-year toxicological study (1991–1995). *Drug Safety* 1997;17:342–356.

14. Boullata JI, Nace AM: Safety issues with herbal medicine. *Pharmacotherapy* 2000;20:257–269.

15. Rivera JO, Ortiz M, Lawson ME, Verma KM: Evaluation of the use of complementary and alternative medicine in the largest United States–Mexico border city. *Pharmacotherapy* 2002;22:256–264.

16. Miller LG: Herbal medicinals: selected clinical considerations focusing on known or potential drug-herb interactions. *Arch Intern Med* 1998;158:220–222.

17. Fugh-Berman A: Herb-drug interactions. *Lancet* 2000;355:134–138.

18. Yuan CS, Wei G, Dey L, et al.: Brief communication: American ginseng reduces warfarin's effect in healthy patients: a randomized, controlled trial. *Ann Intern Med* 2004;141:23–27.

19. Jellin JM, Gregory PJ, Batz F, Hitchens K, et al.: *Pharmacist's Letter/Prescriber's Letter Natural Medicines Comprehensive Database.* 9th ed. Stockton, CA, Therapeutic Research Faculty, 2007.

20. Lee A, Chui PT, Aun CST, Lau ASC, Gin T: Incidence and risk of adverse perioperative events among surgical patients taking traditional Chinese herbal medicines. *Anthesiology* 2006;105:454–461.

21. Ang-Lee MK, Moss J, Yuan CS: Herbal medicines and perioperative care. *JAMA* 2001;286:208–216.

22. Gilroy CM, Steiner JF, Byers T, et al.: Echinacea and truth in labeling. *Arch Intern Med* 2003;163:699–704.

23. Schulz V, Hansel R, Tyler V: *Rational Phytotherapy: A Physician's Guide to Herbal Medicine.* 4th ed. Berlin, Springer-Verlag, 2001.

24. Laakmann G, Schule C, Baghai T, Kieser M: St. John's wort in mild to moderate depression: the relevance of hyperforin for the clinical efficacy. *Pharmacopsychiatry* 1998;31 (Suppl. 1):54–59.

25. Bonati A: How and why should we standardize phytopharmaceutical drugs for clinical validation? *J Ethnopharmacol* 1991;32:195–197.

26. Grant KL: Patient education and herbal dietary supplements. *Am J Health-Syst Pharm* 2000;57:1997–2003.

27. Nortier JL, Muniz Martinez MC, Schmeiser HH, et al.: Urothelial carcinoma associated with the use of a Chinese herb (*Aristolochia fangchi*). *N Engl J Med* 2000;342:1686–1692.

28. Liqiang 4 Dietary Supplement Capsules. Available at http://www.fda.gov/medwatch/SAFETY/2005/safety05.htm#liqiang. Accessed May 21, 2006.

29. Keen RW, Deacon AC, Delves HT, Moreton JA, Frost PG: Indian herbal remedies for diabetes as a cause of lead poisoning. *Postgrad Med J* 1994;70:113–114.

30. Beigel Y, Ostfeld I, Schoenfeld N: Clinical problem-solving: a leading question. *N Engl J Med* 1998;339:827–830.

31. Krochmal R, Hardy M, Bowerman S, et al.: Phytochemical assays of commercial botanical dietary supplements. *ECAM* 2004;1:305–313.

32. Garrard J, Harms S, Eberly LE, Matiak A: Variations in product choices of frequently purchased herbs. *Arch Intern Med* 2003;163:2290–2995.

33. Gill GV, Redmond S, Garratt F, Paisey R: Diabetes and alternative medicine: cause for concern. *Diabet Med* 1994;11:210–213.

34. Garrow D, Egede LE: Association between complementary and alternative medicine use, preventive care practices, and use of conventional medical services among adults with diabetes. *Diabetes Care* 2006;29:15–19.

35. Kaufman DW, Kelly JP, Rosenberg L, Anderson TE, Mitchell AA: Recent patterns of medication use in the ambulatory adult population of the United States. *JAMA* 2002;287:337–344.

36. Leese GP, Gill GV, Houghton GM: Prevalence of complementary medicine usage within a diabetes clinic. *Pract Diab Int* 1997;14:207–208.

37. Ryan EA, Pick ME, Marceau C: Use of alternative medicines in diabetes mellitus. *Diabet Med* 2001;218:242–245.

38. Yeh GY, Eisenberg DM, Davis RB, Phillips RS: Use of complementary and alternative medicine among persons with diabetes mellitus: results of a national survey. *Am J Public Health* 2002;92:1648–1652.

39. Kim C, Kwok YS: Navajo use of native healers. *Arch Intern Med* 1998;158:2245–2249.

40. Noel PH, Pugh JA, Larme AC, Marsh G: The use of traditional plant medicines for non-insulin dependent diabetes mellitus in South Texas. *Phytother Res* 1997;11:512–517.

41. Mull DS, Nguyen N, Mull JD: Vietnamese diabetic patients and their physicians: what ethnography can teach us. *West J Med* 2001;175:307–311.

42. Poss JE, Jezewski MA, Stuart AG: Home remedies for type 2 diabetes used by Mexican Americans in El Paso, Texas. *Clin Nurs Res* 2003;12:304–323.

43. Brown SA, Hanis CL: Culturally competent diabetes education for Mexican Americans: The Starr County study. *Diab Educ* 1999;25:226–236.

44. Ball SD, Kertesz D, Moyer-Mileur LJ: Dietary supplement use is prevalent among children with a chronic illness. *J Am Diet Assoc* 2005;105:78–84.

45. Schoenberg NE, Stoller EP, Kart CS, et al.: Complementary and alternative medicine use among a multiethnic sample of older adults with diabetes. *J Altern Complement Med* 2004;10:1061–1066.

46. Gordon NP, Schaffer DM: Use of dietary supplements by female seniors in a large Northern California health plan. *BMC Geriatrics* 2005;5:4. doi: 10.1186/1471-2318-5-4. (Also available at http://www.biomedcentral. com/1471-2318/5/4)

47. U.S. Food and Drug Administration: Regulation on statements made for dietary supplements concerning the effect of the product on the structure or function of the body. *Fed Register* 2000;65:1000–1050.

48. Wood DM, Athwal S, Panahloo A: The advantages and disadvantages of a 'herbal' medicine in a patient with diabetes mellitus: a case report. *Diabet Med* 2004;21:625–627.

49. U.S. Food and Drug Administration, Center for Food Safety and Applied Nutrition: Dietary supplement strategy (ten-year plan). January 2000. Available at http://vm.cfsan.fda.gov/~dms/ds-strat.html. Accessed May 21, 2006.

50. Harris Poll. *Health Care News* 2002;December 23, Volume 2, Issue 23.

51. U.S. Food and Drug Administration, Center for Food Safety and Applied Nutrition, Office of Nutritional Products, Labeling, and Dietary Supplements: Claims that can be made for conventional foods and dietary supplements. September 2003. Available at http://cfsan.fda.gov/~dms/ hclaims.html. Accessed May 21, 2006.

52. U.S. Pharmacopeia: USP dietary supplement verification program overview. Available at http://www.USP-DSVP.org. Accessed May 21, 2006.

53. NSF International: NSF certified dietary supplements. Available at http://www.nsf.org/certified/dietary/. Accessed May 21, 2006.

54. ConsumerLab.com. Available at http://www.consumerlab.com. Accessed May 21, 2006.

55. Peterson A: New seals of approval certify unregulated herbs, vitamins. *Wall Street Journal* July 10, 2002. Available at http://online.wsj.com/article/0,,SB1026244396762358880.djm,00.html. Accessed January 21, 2007.

56. Herbal Rx: the promises and pitfalls. What's in this stuff? *Consum Rep* 1999; Mar 64:44–48.

57. National Products Association. Available at http://www.naturalproducts assoc.org. Accessed August 31, 2006.

58. Kurtzweil *P:* How to spot health fraud. *FDA Consumer Magazine* November–December 1999. Available at www.fda.gov/fdac/features/1999/699_fraud.html. Accessed May 21, 2006.

59. U.S. Food and Drug Administration, Center for Food Safety and Applied Nutrition, Office of Nutritional Products, Labeling, and Dietary Supplements: Tips for the savvy supplement user: making informed decisions and evaluating information. January 2002. Available at http://www.cfsan.fda.gov/~dms/ds-savvy.html. Accessed May 21, 2006.

60. U.S. Food and Drug Administration, Center for Food Safety and Applied Nutrition, Office of Nutritional Products, Labeling, and Dietary Supplements: Tips for older dietary supplement users. December 2003. Available at http://www.cfsan.fda.gov/~dms/ds-savv2.html Accessed May 21, 2006.

61. Sarubin Fragakis A: *The Health Professional's Guide to Popular Dietary Supplements.* 2nd ed. Chicago, American Dietetic Association, 2003.

62. Blumenthal M, Busse WR, Goldberg A, et al. (Eds.): *The Complete German Commission E Monographs: Therapeutic Guide to Herbal Medicines.* Klein S, trans. Boston, American Botanical Council, 1998.

63. The Epicentre: Encyclopedia of spices: cassia (*Cinnamomum cassia*). Available at http://www.theepicentre.com/Spices/cassia.html. Accessed September 9, 2004.

64. Jarvill-Taylor KJ, Anderson RA, Graves DJ: A hydroxychalcone derived from cinnamon functions as a mimetic for insulin in 3T3-L1 adipocytes. *J Am Coll Nutr* 2001;20:327–336.

65. Khan A, Safdar M, Ali Khan MM, et al.: Cinnamon improves glucose and lipids of people with type 2 diabetes. *Diabetes Care* 2003;26:3215–3218.

66. Mang B, Wolters M, Schmitt B, et al.: Effects of a cinnamon extract on plasma glucose, HbA1c, and serum lipids in diabetes mellitus type 2. *Eur J Clin Invest* 2006;36:340–344.

67. Yoshikawa M, Murakami T, Kadoya M, et al.: Medicinal foodstuffs. IX. The inhibitors of glucose absorption from the leaves of *Gymnema sylvestre* R. Br. (*Asclepiadaceae*): structures of gymnemosides a and b. *Chem Pharm Bull* 1997;45:1671–1676.

68. Anonymous: *Gymnema sylvestre. Altern Med Rev* 1999;4:46–47.

69. Shanmugasundaram ERB, Rajeswari G, Baskaran K, et al.: Use of *Gymnema sylvestre* leaf extract in the control of blood glucose in insulin-dependent diabetes mellitus. *J Ethnopharmacol* 1990;30:281–294.

70. Kapoor LD: *Handbook of Ayurvedic Medicinal Plants.* Boca Raton, Fla., CRC Press, 1990, pp. 200–201.

71. Shanmugasundaram ER, Panneerselvam C, Samudram P, Shanmugasundaram ERB: Enzyme changes and glucose utilization in diabetic rabbits: the effect of *Gymnema sylvestre. J Ethnopharmacol* 1983;7:205–234.

72. Persaud SJ, Al-Majed H, Raman A, Jones PM: *Gymnema sylvestre* stimulates insulin release in vitro by increased membrane permeability. *J Endocrinol* 1999;163:207–212.

73. Shanmugasundaram ERB, Gopinath KL, Shanmugasundaram KR, Rajendran VM: Possible regeneration of the islets of Langerhans in streptozotocin-diabetic rats given *Gymnema sylvestre* leaf extracts. *J Ethnopharmacol* 1990;30:265–279.

74. Baskaran K, Kizar B, Ahamath K, et al.: Antidiabetic effect of a leaf extract from *Gymnema sylvestre* in non-insulin-dependent diabetes mellitus patients. *J Ethnopharmacol* 1990;30:295–306.

75. DerMarderosian A, Beutler JA (Eds.): *The Review of Natural Products.* St. Louis, Mo., Wolters Kluwer Health, 2006.

76. Patil SP, Niphadkar PV, Bapat MM: Allergy to fenugreek (*Trigonella foenum graecum*). *Ann Allergy Asthma Immunol* 1997;78:297–300.

77. Madar Z: Fenugreek (*Trigonella foenum-graeceum*) as a means of reducing postprandial glucose levels in diabetic rats. *Nutr Rep Int* 1984;23:1267–1273.

78. Raghuram TC, Sharma R, Sivakumar D, Sahay BK: Effect of fenugreek seeds on intravenous glucose disposition in non-insulin dependent diabetic patients. *Phytotherapy Res* 1994;8:83–86.

79. Flammang AM, Cifone MA, Erexson GL, Stankowski LF Jr: Genotoxicity testing of a fenugreek extract. *Food Chem Toxicol* 2004;42:1769–1775.

80. Lambert J, Cormier J: Potential interaction between warfarin and boldofenugreek. *Pharmacotherapy* 2001;21:509–512.

81. Sharma RD, Raghuram TC, Sudhakar Rao N: Effect of fenugreek seeds on blood glucose and serum lipids in type 1 diabetes. *Eur J Clin Nutr* 1990;44:301–306.

82. Sharma RD, Sarkar A, Hazra DK, et al.: Use of fenugreek seed powder in the management of non-insulin-dependent diabetes mellitus. *Nutr Res* 1996;16:1331–1339.

83. Gupta A, Gupta R, Lal B: Effect of *Trigonella foenum-graecum* (fenugreek) seeds on glycaemic control and insulin resistance in type 2 diabetes mellitus: a double blind placebo controlled study. *J Assoc Physicians India* 2001;49:1057–1061.

84. U.S. Food and Drug Administration, Center for Food Safety and Applied Nutrition: EAFUS: A food additive database. Available at http://vm.cfsan.fda.gov/~dms/eafus.html. Accessed May 29, 2006.

85. Basch E, Gabardi S, Ulbricht C: Bitter melon (*Momordica charantia*): a review of efficacy and safety. *Am J Health-Syst Pharm* 2003;60:356–359.

86. Bitter melon, bitter gourd (*Momordica charantia*). Available at http://www.intelihealth.com. Accessed March 29, 2007.

87. Aslam M, Stockley IH: Interaction between curry ingredient (karela) and drug (chlorpropamide) (Letter). *Lancet* 1979;1:607.

88. Ahmad N, Hassan MR, Halder H, Bennoor KS: Effect of *Momordica charantia* (karolla) extracts on fasting and postprandial serum glucose levels in NIDDM patients. *Bangladesh Med Res Counc Bull* 1999;25:11–13.

89. Khanna P, Jain SC, Panagariya A, Dixit VP: Hypoglycemic activity of polypeptide-p from a plant source. *J Nat Prod* 1981;44:648–655.

90. Srivastava Y, Venkatakrishna-Bhatt H, Verma Y, Venkaiah K: Antidiabetic and adaptogenic properties of *Momordica charantia* extract: an experimental and clinical evaluation. *Phytother Res* 1993;7:285–289.

91. Kiefer D, Pantuso T: *Panax ginseng*. *Am Fam Physician* 2003;68:1539–1542.

92. Vuksan V, Sievenpiper JL, Koo VYY, Francis T, Beljan-Zdravkovic U, Xu Z, Vidgen E: American ginseng (*Panax quinquefolius* L.) reduces postprandial glycemia in nondiabetic subjects and subjects with type 2 diabetes mellitus. *Arch Intern Med* 2000;160:1009–1013.

93. Hong B, Ji YH, Hong JH, Nam KY, Ahn TY: A double-blind crossover study evaluating the efficacy of Korean red ginseng in patients with erectile dysfunction: a preliminary report. *J Urol* 2002;168:2070–2073.

94. Raman A, Houston P: Herbal products: ginseng. *Pharm J* 1995;255:150–152.

95. Yuan CS, Wu JA, Lowell T, Gu M: Gut and brain effects of American ginseng root on brain-stem neuronal activities in rats. *Am J Chin Med* 1998;26:47–55.

96. Ohnishi Y, Takagi S, Miura T, et al.: Effect of ginseng radix on GLUT2 protein content in mouse liver in normal and epinephrine-induced hyperglycemic mice. *Biol Pharm Bull* 1996;19:1238–1240.

97. Kimura M, Waki I, Chujo T, et al.: Effects of hypoglycemic components in ginseng radix on blood insulin level in alloxan diabetic mice and on insulin release from perfused rat pancreas. *J Pharmacobiodyn* 1981;4:410–417.

98. Vuksan V, Stavro MP, Sievenpiper JL, et al.: Similar postprandial glycemic reductions with escalation of dose and administration time of American ginseng in type 2 diabetes. *Diabetes Care* 2000;23:1221–1226.

99. Sotaniemi EA, Haapakoski E, Rautio A: Ginseng therapy in non-insulin dependent diabetic patients. *Diabetes Care* 1995;18:1373–1375.

100. Harkey MR, Henderson GL, Gershwin ME, Stern JS, Hacman RM: Variability in commercial ginseng products: an analysis of 25 preparations. *Am J Clin Nutr* 2001;73:1101–1106.

101. Cui J, Garle M, Eneroth P, Bjorkhem I: What do commercial ginseng preparations contain? (Letter). *Lancet* 1994;344:134.

102. Wiese J, McPherson S, Odden MC, Shlipak MG: Effect of *Opuntia ficus indica* on symptoms of the alcohol hangover. *Arch Intern Med* 2004;164:1334–1340.

103. Palevitch D, Earon G, Levin I: Treatment of benign prostatic hypertrophy with *Opuntia ficus-indica* (L.) Miller. *Int J Comp Alt Med* 1994;Sept.:21–22.

104. Ibanez-Camacho R, Roman-Ramos R: Hypoglycemic effect of *Opuntia* cactus. *Arch Invest Med* 1979;10:223–230.

105. Rayburn K, Martinez R, Escobedo M, et al.: Glycemic effects of various species of nopal (*Opuntia* sp.) in type 2 diabetes mellitus. *Texas J Rural Health* 1998;26:68–76.

106. Meckes-Lozyoa M, Roman-Ramos R: *Opuntia streptacantha*: a coajutor in the treatment of diabetes mellitus. *Am J Chin Med* 1986;14:116–118.

107. Frati-Munari AC, Gordillo BE, Altamirano P, Ariza CR: Hypoglycemic effect of *Opuntia streptacantha* Lemaire in NIDDM. *Diabetes Care* 1988;11:63–66.

108. Frati AC, Gordillo BE, Altamirano P, Ariza CR, Cortes-Franco R, Chavez-Negrete A: Acute hypoglycemic effect of *Opuntia streptacantha* Lemaire in NIDDM (Letter). *Diabetes Care* 1990;13:45–46.

109. Yongchaiyudha S, Rungpitarangsi V, Bunyapraphatsara N, Chokechai-jaroenporn O: Antidiabetic activity of *Aloe vera* L. juice. I. Clinical trial in new cases of diabetes mellitus. *Phytomedicine* 1996;3:241–243.

110. Bunyapraphatsara N, Yongchaiyudha S, Rungpitarangsi Chokechaijaroen-porn O: Antidiabetic activity of *Aloe vera* L. juice. II. Clinical trial in diabetes mellitus patients in combination with glibenclamide. *Phytomedicine* 1996;3:245–248.

111. Lee A, Chui PT, Aun CST, et al.: Possible interaction between sevoflurance and *Aloe vera*. *Ann Pharmacother* 2004;38:1651–1654.

112. Ghannam N: The antidiabetic activity of aloes: preliminary clinical and experimental observations. *Horm Res* 1986;24:288–294.

113. Judy WV, Hari SP, Stogsdill WW, et al.: Antidiabetic activity of a standardized extract (Glucosol^{TM}) from *Lagerstroemia speciosa* leaves in type II diabetics: a dose-dependence study. *J Ethnopharmacol* 2003;87:115–117.

114. Hayashi T, Maruyama H, Kasai R, et al.: Ellagitannins from *Lagerstroemia speciosa* as activators of glucose transport in fat cells. *Planta Med* 2002;68:173–175.

115. Hattori K, Sukenobu N, Sasaki T, et al.: Activation of insulin receptors by lagerstroemin. *J Pharmacol Sci* 2003;93:69–73.

116. Ludvik B, Neuffer B, Pacini G: Efficacy of *Ipomoea batatas* (caiapo) on diabetes control in type 2 diabetic subjects treated with diet. *Diabetes Care* 2004;27:436–440.

117. Ludvik B, Waldhausl W, Prager R, et al.: Mode of action of *Ipomoea batatas* (caiapo) in type 2 diabetic patients. *Metabolism* 2003;52:875–880.

118. Kusano S, Abe H, Tamura H: Isolation of antidiabetic components from white-skinned sweet potato (*Ipomoea batatas* L.). *Biosci Biotechnol Biochem* 2001;65:109–114.

119. Ludvik BH, Mahdjoobian K, Waldhausl W, et al.: The effect of *Ipomoea batatas* (caiapo) on glucose metabolism and serum cholesterol in patients with type 2 diabetes. *Diabetes Care* 2002;25:239–240.

120. Wasantwisut E, Viriyapanich T: Ivy gourd (*Coccinia grandis* Voigt, *Coccinia cordifolia, Coccinia indica*) in human nutrition and traditional applications. *World Rev Nutr Diet* 2003;91:60–66.

121. Azad Khan AK, Akhtar S, Mahtab H: *Coccinia indica* in the treatment of patients with diabetes mellitus. *Bangladesh Med Res Council Bull* 1979;5:60–66.

122. Kamble SM, Kamlakar PL, Vaidya S, Bambole VD: Influence of *Coccinia indica* on certain enzymes in glycolytic and lipolytic pathway in human diabetes. *Indian J Med Sci* 1998;52:143–146.

123. Kamble SM, Jyotishi GS, Kamlakar PL, Vaidya SM: Efficacy of *Coccinia indica* S & A in diabetes mellitus. *J Res Ayurveda Siddha* 1996;XVII:77–84.

124. Fetrow CW, Avila JR (Eds.): *Professional's Handbook of Complementary and Alternative Medicines.* 3rd ed. Springhouse, PA, Lippincott Williams & Wilkins, 2004.

125. Godhwani S, Godhwani JL, Vyas DS: *Ocimum sanctum*: an experimental study evaluating its anti-inflammatory, analgesic and antipyretic activity in animals. *J Ethnopharmacol* 1987;21:153–163.

126. Khanna N, Bhatia J: Antinociceptive action of *Ocimum sanctum* (Tulsi) in mice: possible mechanisms involved. *J Ethnopharmacol* 2003;88:293–296.

127. Agrawal P, Rai V, Singh RB: Randomized placebo-controlled, single blind trial of holy basil leaves in patients with noninsulin-dependent diabetes mellitus. *Int J Clin Pharmacol Ther* 1996;34:406–409.

128. Seth SD, Johri N, Sundaram KR: Antispermatogenic effect of *Ocimum sanctum. Indian J Exp Biol* 1981;19:975–976.

129. Kasinathan S, Ramakrishnan S, Basu SL: Antifertility effect of *Ocimum sanctum* L. *Indian J Exp Biol* 1972;10:23–25.

130. Singh S, Rehan HM, Majumdar DK: Effect of *Ocimum sanctum* fixed oil on blood pressure, blood clotting time and pentobarbitone-induced sleeping time. *J Ethnopharmacol* 2001;78:139–143.

131. Dhanabal SP, Kokate CK, Ramanathan M, et al.: Hypoglycaemic activity of *Pterocarpus marsupium* Roxb. *Phytother Res* 2006;20:4–8.

132. Jung M, Park M, Lee HC, et al.: Antidiabetic agents from medicinal plants. *Curr Med Chem* 2006;13:1203–1218.

133. Saxena A, Vikram NK: Role of selected Indian plants in the management of type 2 diabetes: a review. *J Altern Complement Med* 2004;10:369–378.

134. Indian Council of Medical Research: Flexible dose open trail of Vijayasar in cases of newly diagnosed non-insulin dependent diabetes mellitus. *Indian J Med Res* 1998;108:24–29.

135. Morton J: Jambolan. In *Fruits of warm climates*. Miami, Fla., Julia F. Morton, 1987, pp. 375–378. Available at http://www.hort.purdue.edu/newcrop/morton/jambolan.html. Accessed July 8, 2006.

136. Teixeira CC, Weinert LS, Barbosa DC, et al.: *Syzygium cumini* (L.) Skeels in the treatment of type 2 diabetes. *Diabetes Care* 2004;27:3019–3020.

137. Teixeira CC, Fuchs FD, Weinert LS, Esteves J: The efficacy of folk medicines in the management of type 2 diabetes mellitus: results of a randomized controlled trial of *Syzygium cumini* (L.) Skeels. *J Pharmacol Ther* 2006;31:1–5.

138. Kohli KR, Singh RH: A clinical trial of jambu (*Eugenia jambolana*) in non-insulin dependent diabetes mellitus. *J Res Ayurveda Sidda* 1993;14:89–97.

139. Sierra M, Garcia JJ, Fernandez N, et al.: Therapeutic effects of psyllium in type 2 diabetic patients. *Eur J Clin Nutr* 2002;56:830–842.

140. Gruenwald J, Brendler T, Jaenicke C (Eds.): *PDR for Herbal Medicines*. 2nd ed. Montvale, NJ, Thomson Medical Economics, 2000.

141. Pastors JG, Blaisdell PW, Balm TK, et al.: Psyllium fiber reduces rise in postprandial glucose and insulin concentrations in patients with non-insulin-dependent diabetes. *Am J Clin Nutr* 1991;53:1431–1435.

142. Rodriguez-Moran M, Guerrero-Romero F, Lazcano-Burciaga G: Lipid and glucose lowering efficacy of plantago psyllium in type II diabetes. *J Diabetes Complications* 1998;12:273–278.

143. Anderson JW, Allgood LD, Turner J, et al.: Effects of psyllium on glucose and serum lipid responses in men with type 2 diabetes and hypercholesterolemia. *Am J Clin Nutr* 1999;70:466–473.

144. Metamucil. Available at www.metamucil.com. Accessed July 11, 2006.

145. U.S. Food and Drug Administration: FDA Talk Paper: FDA allows foods containing psyllium to make health claim on reducing risk of heart disease. February 1998. Available at http://www.fda.gov/bbs/topics/ANSWERS/ANS00850.html. Accessed July 11, 2006.

146. Chen HL, Sheu WH-H, Tai T-S, et al.: Konjac supplement alleviated hypercholesterolemia and hyperglycemia in type 2 diabetic subjects: a randomized double-blind trial. *J Am Coll Nutr* 2003;22:36–42.

147. Vuksan V, Jenkins DJA, Spadafora P, et al.: Konjac-mannan (glucomannan) improves glycemia and other associated risk factors for coronary heart disease in type 2 diabetes, a randomized controlled metabolic trial. *Diabetes Care* 1999;22:913–919.

148. Vuksan V, Sievenpiper JL, Owen R, et al.: Beneficial effects of viscous dietary fiber from konjac-mannan in subjects with the insulin resistance syndrome, results of a controlled metabolic trial. *Diabetes Care* 2000;23:9–14.

149. Huang CY, Zhang MY, Peng SS, et al.: Effect of konjac food on blood glucose level in patients with diabetes. *Biomed Environ Sci* 1990;3:123–131.

150. Uusitupa MI, Miettinen TA, Happonen P, et al.: Lathosterol and other noncholesterol sterols during treatment of hypercholesterolemia with lovastatin alone and with cholestyramine or guar gum. *Arterioscler Throm* 1992;12:807–813.

151. Vuorinen-Markkola H, Sinisalo M, Koivisto VA: Guar gum in insulin-dependent diabetes: effects on glycemic control and serum lipoproteins. *Am J Clin Nutr* 1991;56:1056–1060.

152. Groop PH, Aro A, Stenman S, Groop L: Long-term effects of guar gum in subjects with non-insulin-dependent diabetes mellitus. *Am J Clin Nutr* 1993;58:513–518.

153. Pittler MH, Ernst E: Guar gum for body weight reduction: meta-analysis of randomized trials. *Am J Med* 2001;110:724–730.

154. Kirsten R, Heintz B, Nelson K, Oremek G, Speck U: Influence of two guar preparations on glycosylated hemoglobin, total cholesterol and

triglycerides in patients with diabetes mellitus. *Int J Clin Pharmacol Ther Toxicol* 1992;30:582–586.

155. Hsieh M-H, Chan P, Sue Y-M, et al.: Efficacy and tolerability of oral stevioside in patients with mild essential hypertension: a two-year, randomized, placebo-controlled study. *Clin Ther* 2003;25:2797–2808.

156. Anonymous: More about stevia, a non-approved sweetener. *Harv Womens Health Watch* 2005;12:6–7.

157. Curi R, Alvarez M, Bazotte RB, et al.: Effect of *Stevia rebaudiana* on glucose tolerance in normal adult humans. *Braz J Med Biol Res* 1986;19:771–774.

158. Jeppesen PB, Gregersen S, Poulsen CR, Hermansen K: Stevioside acts directly on pancreatic beta cells to secrete insulin: actions independent of cyclic adenosine monophosphate and adenosine triphosphate-sensitive K+-channel activity. *Metabolism* 2000;49:208–214.

159. Gregersen S, Jeppesen PB, Holst JJ, Hermansen K: Antihyperglycemic effects of stevioside in type 2 diabetic subjects. *Metabolism* 2004;53:73–76.

160. Chan P, Tomlinson B, Chen Y-J, et al.: A double-blind placebo-controlled study of the effectiveness and tolerability of oral stevioside in human hypertension. *Br J Clin Pharmacol* 2000;50:215–220.

161. Rohdewald P: A review of the French maritime pine bark extract (Pycnogenol®), a herbal medication with a diverse clinical pharmacology. *Int J Clin Pharmacol Ther* 2002;40:158–168.

162. Spadea L, Balestrazzi E: Treatment of vascular retinopathy with Pycnogenol®. *Phytother Res* 2001;15:219–223.

163. Liu X, Zhou H-J, Rohdewald P: French maritime pine bark extract Pycnogenol dose-dependently lowers glucose in type 2 diabetes patients (Letter). *Diabetes Care* 2004;27:839.

164. Schonlau F, Rohdewald P: Pycnogenol® for diabetic retinopathy. *Int Ophthalmology* 2001;24:161–171.

165. Liu X, Wei J, Tan F, et al.: Antidiabetic effect of Pycnogenol® French maritime pine bark extract in patients with diabetes type II. *Life Sci* 2004;75:2505–2513.

166. Anonymous: Green tea. *Altern Med Rev* 2000;5:372–375.

167. Hosoda K, Wang MF, Liao ML, et al.: Antihyperglycemic effect of oolong tea in type 2 diabetes. *Diabetes Care* 2003;26:1714–1718.

168. Cabrera C, Artacho R, Gimenez R: Beneficial effects of green tea: a review. *J Am Coll Nutr* 2006;25:79–99.

169. Han LK, Takaku K, Li J, et al.: Anti-obesity action of oolong tea. *Int J Obes Relat Metab Disord* 1999;23:98–105.

170. Iso H, Date X, Wakai K, et al.: The relationship between green tea and total caffeine intake and risk for self-reported type 2 diabetes among Japanese adults. *Ann Intern Med* 2006;144:554–562.

171. Anderson RA, Polansky MM: Tea enhances insulin activity. *J Agric Food Chem* 2002;50:8182–8186.

172. Shimada K, Kawarabayashi T, Tanaka A, et al.: Oolong tea increases plasma adiponectin levels and low-density lipoprotein particle size in patients with coronary artery disease. *Diab Res Clin Pract* 2004;65:227–234.

173. Eschenauer G, Sweet BV: Pharmacology and therapeutic uses of theanine. *Am J Health-Syst Pharm* 2006;63:26,28–30.

174. Bonkovsky HL: Hepatotoxicity associated with supplements containing Chinese green tea (*Camellia sinensis*) (Letter). *Ann Intern Med* 2006; 144:68–71

175. Maron DJ, Lu GP, Cai NS, et al.: Cholesterol-lowering effect of a theaflavin-enriched green tea extract: a randomized controlled trial. *Arch Intern Med* 2003;163:1448–1453.

176. Bravetti G: Preventive medical treatment of senile cataract with vitamin E and anthocyanosides: clinical evaluation. *Ann Ottalmol Clin Ocul* 1989;115:109.

177. Cignarella A, Nastasi M, Cavalli E, Puglisi L: Novel lipid-lowering properties of *Vaccinium myrtillus* L. leaves, a traditional antidiabetic treatment, in several models of rat dyslipidaemia: a comparison with ciprofibrate. *Thrombosis Res* 1996;84:311–322.

178. Muth ER, Laurent JM, Jasper P: The effect of bilberry nutritional supplementation on night visual acuity and contrast sensitivity. *Altern Med Rev* 2000;5:164–173.

179. Levy Y, Glovinsky Y: The effect of anthocyanosides on night vision. *Eye* 1998;12:967–969.

180. Zadok D, Levy Y, Glovinsky Y: The effect of anthocyanosides in a multiple oral dose on night vision. *Eye* 1999;13:734–736.

181. Perossini M, Guidi G, Chiellini S, Siravo D: [Diabetic and hypertensive retinopathy therapy with *Vaccinium myrtillus* anthocyanosides (Tegens): Double blind, placebo-controlled clinical trial] [Article in Italian]. *Ann Ottalmol Clin Ocul* 1987;113:1173–1177.

182. Pepping J: Alternative therapies: milk thistle: *Silybum marianum. Am J Health-Syst Pharm* 1999;56:1195–1197.

183. Flora K, Hahn M, Rosen H, Benner K: Milk thistle (*Silybum marinum*) for the therapy of liver disease. *Am J Gastroenterol* 1998;93:139–143.

184. Velussi M, Cernigoi AM, De Monte A, et al.: Long-term (12 months) treatment with an anti-oxidant drug (silymarin) is effective on hyperinsulinemia, exogenous insulin need and malondialdehyde levels in cirrhotic diabetic patients. *J Hepatol* 1997;26:871–879.

185. Rainone F: Milk thistle. *Am Fam Physician* 2005;72:1285–1288.

186. Luper S: A review of plants used in the treatment of liver disease: part 1. *Altern Med Rev* 1998;3:410–421.

187. Adverse Drug Reactions Advisory Committee: An adverse reaction to the herbal medication milk thistle (*Silybum marianum*). *Med J Aust* 1999;170:218–219.

188. Rambaldi A, Jacobs BP, Iaquinto G, Gluud C: Milk thistle for alcoholic and/or hepatitis B or C liver diseases: a systematic Cochrane Hepatobiliary Group review with meta-analyses of randomized clinical trials. *Am J Gastroenterol* 2005;100:2583–2591.

189. Huseini HF, Larijani B, Heshmat R, et al.: The efficacy of *Silybum marianum* (L.) Gaertn. (silymarin) in the treatment of type II diabetes: a randomized, double-blind, placebo-controlled, clinical trial. *Phytother Res* 2006;20:1036–1039.

190. Medina J, Fernandez-Salazar LI, Garcia-Buey L, Moreno-Otero R: Approach to the pathogenesis and treatment of nonalcoholic steatohepatitis. *Diabetes Care* 2004;27:2057–2066.

191. Cefalu WT, Hu FB: Role of chromium in human health and in diabetes. *Diabetes Care* 2004;27:2741–2751.

192. Chavez ML: Chromium picolinate. *Hospital Pharmacy* 1997;32:1466, 1471–1473, 1477–1478.

193. Anderson R, Polansky M, Bryden N, Canary J: Supplemental chromium effects on glucose, insulin, glucagon, and urinary chromium losses in subjects consuming controlled low-chromium diets. *Am J Clin Nutr* 1991;54:909–916.

194. Davidson IWF, Burt RL: Physiologic changes in plasma chromium of normal and pregnant women: effect of a glucose load. *Am J Obstet* 1973;116:601–608.

195. Ravina A, Slezak L, Mirsky N, Bryden NA, Anderson RA: Reversal of corticosteroid-induced diabetes mellitus with supplemental chromium. *Diabet Med* 1999;16:164–167.

196. Food and Nutrition Board, Institute of Medicine: *Dietary Reference Intakes for Vitamin A, Vitamin K, Arsenic, Boron, Chromium, Copper, Iodine, Iron, Manganese, Molybdenum, Nickel, Silicon, Vanadium, and Zinc.* Washington, D.C., National Academy Press, 2000. Available at www.nap.edu/books/0309072794/html. Accessed July 30, 2006.

197. Wasser WG, Feldman NS, D'Agati VD: Chronic renal failure after ingestion of over the counter chromium picolinate (Letter). *Ann Intern Med* 1997;126:410.

198. Cerulli J, Grabe DW, Gauthier I, Malone M, McGoldrick MD: Chromium picolinate toxicity. *Ann Pharmacotherapy* 1998;32:428–431.

199. Martin WR, Fuller RE: Suspected chromium picolinate-induced rhabdomyolysis. *Pharmacotherapy* 1998;18:860–862.

200. Young PC, Turiansky GW, Bonner MW, Benson PM: Acute generalized exanthematous pustulosis induced by chromium picolinate. *J Am Acad Dermatol* 1999;41:820–823.

201. Anderson RA, Cheng N, Bryden NA, et al.: Elevated intakes of supplemental chromium improves glucose and insulin variables in individuals with type 2 diabetes. *Diabetes* 1997;46:1786–1791.

202. Jeejeebhoy KN: The role of chromium in nutrition and therapeutics and as a potential toxin. *Nutr Rev* 1999;57:329–335.

203. Rajpathak S, Rimm EB, Li T, et al.: Lower toenail chromium in men with diabetes and cardiovascular disease compared with healthy men. *Diabetes Care* 2004;27:2211–2216.

204. Althuis MD, Jordan NE, Ludington EA, Wittes JT: Glucose and insulin responses to dietary chromium supplements: a meta analysis. *Am J Clin Nutr* 2002;76:148–155.

205. Gunton JE, Cheung NW, Hitchman R, et al.: Chromium supplementation does not improve glucose tolerance, insulin sensitivity, or lipid profile: a randomized, placebo-controlled, double-blind trial of supplementation in subjects with impaired glucose tolerance. *Diabetes Care* 2005;28:712–713.

206. Kleefstra N, Houweling S, Jansman FGA, et al.: Chromium treatment has no effect in patients with poorly controlled, insulin-treated type 2 diabetes

in an obese Western population: a randomized, double-blind, placebo-controlled trial. *Diabetes Care* 2006;29:521–525.

207. Komorowski J, Juturu V: Chromium supplementation does not improve glucose tolerance, insulin sensitivity, or lipid profile: a randomized, placebo-controlled, double-blind trial of supplementation in subjects with impaired glucose tolerance: response to Gunton et al. (Letter). *Diabetes Care* 2005;28:1841–1842; author reply 1842–1843.

208. Diachrome. Available at www.diachrome.com. Accessed July 30, 2006.

209. U.S. Food and Drug Administration, Center for Food Safety and Applied Nutrition, Office of Nutritional Products, Labeling, and Dietary Supplements: Qualified health claims: letter of enforcement discretion: chromium picolinate and insulin resistance. Docket No. 2004Q-0144. Available at http://www.cfsan.fda.gov/~dms/qhccr.html. Accessed July 30, 2006.

210. Cefalu WT, Bell-Farrow AD, Stegner J, et al.: Effect of chromium picolinate on insulin sensitivity in vivo. *J Trace Elem Exp Med* 1999;12:71–83.

211. American Diabetes Association: Nutrition principles and recommendations in diabetes (Position Statement). *Diabetes Care* 2004;27 (Suppl. 1):S36–S46.

212. Srivastava AK, Mehdi MZ: Insulino-mimetic and anti-diabetic effects of vanadium compounds. *Diabet Med* 2005;22:2–13.

213. Poucheret P, Verma S, Grynpas MD, et al.: Vanadium and diabetes. *Mol Cell Biochem* 1998;188:73–80.

214. Fawcett JP, Farquhar SJ, Walker RJ, Thou T, Lowe G, Goulding A: The effect of oral vanadyl sulfate on body composition and performance in weight-training athletes. *Int J Sport Nutr* 1996;6:382–390.

215. Fantus IG, Tsiani E: Multifunctional actions of vanadium compounds on insulin signaling pathways: evidence for preferential enhancement of metabolic versus mitogenic effects. *Mol Cell Biochem* 1998;182:109–119.

216. Cohen N, Halberstam M, Shlimovich P, Chang CJ, Shamoon H, Rossetti L: Oral vanadyl sulfate improves hepatic and peripheral insulin sensitivity in patients with non-insulin-dependent diabetes mellitus. *J Clin Invest* 1995;95:2501–2509.

217. Swarup G, Cohen S, Garbers DL: Inhibition of membrane phosphotyrosyl-protein phosphatase activity by vanadate. *Biochem Biophys Res Comm* 1982;107:1104–1109.

218. Domingo JL, Gomez M, Llobet JM, Corbella J, Keen CL: Oral vanadium administration to streptozotocin-diabetic rats has marked negative side effects which are independent of the form of vanadium used. *Toxicology* 1991;66:279–287.

219. Carpenter G: Vanadate, epidermal growth factor and the stimulation of DNA synthesis. *Biochem Biophys Res Comm* 1981;102:1115–1121.

220. Klarlund JK: Transformation of cells by an inhibitor of phosphatases acting on phosphotyrosine in proteins. *Cell* 1985;41:707–717.

221. Naylor GJ, Smith AH: Vanadium: a possible aetiological factor in manic depressive illness. *Psychol Med* 1981;11:249–256.

222. Funakoshi T, Shimada H, Kojima S, et al.: Anticoagulant action of vanadate. *Chem Pharm Bull* 1992;40:174–176.

223. Goldfine AB, Simonson DC, Folli F, Patti ME, Kahn CR: Metabolic effects of sodium metavanadate in humans with insulin-dependent and non-insulin-dependent diabetes mellitus: in vivo and in vitro studies. *J Clin Endocrinol Metab* 1995;80:3311–3320.

224. Boden G, Chen X, Ruiz J, van Rossum GDV, Turco S: Effects of vanadyl sulfate on carbohydrate and lipid metabolism in patients with non-insulin dependent diabetes mellitus. *Metabolism* 1996;45:1130–1135.

225. Goldfine AB, Patti ME, Zuberi L, et al.: Metabolic effects of vanadyl sulfate in humans with non-insulin-dependent diabetes mellitus: in vivo and in vitro studies. Metabolism 2000;49:400–410.

226. Elliott RB, Pilcher CC, Fergusson DM, et al.: A population-based strategy to prevent insulin-dependent diabetes using nicotinamide. *J Pediatr Endocrinol Metab* 1996;501–509.

227. Pozilli P, Browne PD, Kolb H, the Nicotinamide Trialists: Meta-analysis of nicotinamide treatment in patients with recent-onset IDDM. *Diabetes Care* 1996;19:1357–1363.

228. Polo V, Saibene A, Pontiroli AE: Nicotinamide improves insulin secretion and metabolic control in lean type 2 diabetic patients with secondary failure to sulphonylureas. *Acta Diabetol* 1998;35:61–64.

229. Head KA: Type-1 diabetes: prevention of the disease and its complications. *Altern Med Rev* 1997;2:256–281.

230. Bourgeois BFD, Dodson WE, Ferrendelli JA: Interactions between primidone, carbamazepine, and nicotinamide. *Neurology* 1982;32:1122–1126.

231. Gale EA, Bingley PJ, Emmett CL, Collier T, European Nicotinamide Diabetes Intervention Trial (ENDIT) Group: European Nicotinamide Diabetes Intervention Trial (ENDIT): a randomized controlled trial of intervention before the onset of type 1 diabetes. *Lancet* 2004;363:925–931.

232. Crino A, Schiaffini R, Manfrini S, et al.: A randomized trial of nicotinamide and vitamin E in children with recent onset type 1 diabetes (IMDIAB IX). *Eur J Endocrinol* 2004;150:719–724.

233. Crino A, Schiaffini R, Ciampalini P, et al.: A two year observational study of nicotinamide and intensive insulin therapy in patients with recent onset type 1 diabetes mellitus. *J Pediatr Endocrinol Metab* 2005;18:749–754.

234. Guerrero-Romero F, Rodriguez-Moran M: Complementary therapies for diabetes: the case for chromium, magnesium, and antioxidants. *Arch Med Res* 2005;36:150–157.

235. Lopez-Ridaura R, Willett WC, Rimm EB, et al.: Magnesium intake and risk of type 2 diabetes in men and women. *Diabetes Care* 2004;27:134–140.

236. Pereira MA, Parker ED, Folsom AR: Coffee consumption and risk of type 2 diabetes mellitus. *Arch Intern Med* 2006;166:1311–1316.

237. Bruinsma K, Taren DL: Chocolate: food or drug? *J Am Diet Assoc* 1999;99:1249–1256.

238. deLourdes Lima M, Cruz T, Pousada JC, et al.: The effect of magnesium supplementation in increasing doses on the control of type 2 diabetes. *Diabetes Care* 1998;21:682–686.

239. Rodriguez-Moran M, Guerrero-Romero F: Low serum magnesium levels and foot ulcers in subjects with type 2 diabetes. *Arch Med Res* 2001;32:300–303.

240. Kao WHL, Folsom AR, Nieto FJ, et al.: Serum and dietary magnesium and the risk for type 2 diabetes mellitus, the atherosclerosis risk in communities study. *Arch Intern Med* 1999;159:2151–2159.

241. Rodriguez-Moran M, Guerrero-Romero F: Oral magnesium supplementation improves insulin sensitivity and metabolic control in type 2 diabetes subjects. *Diabetes Care* 2003;26:1147–1153.

242. Eibl NL, Kopp H-P, Nowak HR, et al.: Hypomagnesemia in type II diabetes: effect of a 3-month replacement therapy. *Diabetes Care* 1995;18:188–192.

243. de Valk HW, Verkaaik R, van Rijn HJM, et al.: Oral magnesium supplementation in insulin-requiring type 2 diabetic patients. *Diabet Med* 1998;15:503–507.

244. American Diabetes Association: Magnesium supplementation in the treatment of diabetes (Consensus Statement). *Diabetes Care* 1992;15:1065–1067.

245. Bonakdar RA, Guarneri E: Coenzyme Q10. *Am Fam Physician* 2005;72:1065–1070.

246. Tran MT, Mitchell TM, Kennedy DT, Giles JT: Role of coenzyme Q10 in chronic heart failure, angina, and hypertension. *Pharmacotherapy* 2001;21:797–806.

247. Pepping J: Alternative therapies: coenzyme Q10. *Am J Health-Syst Pharm* 1999;56:519–521.

248. Gaby AR: The role of coenzyme Q10 in clinical medicine. II. Cardiovascular disease, hypertension, diabetes mellitus and infertility. *Altern Med Rev* 1996;1:168–175.

249. McCarty MF: Can correction of sub-optimal coenzyme Q status improve β-cell function in type II diabetics? *Med Hypotheses* 1999;52:397–400.

250. Langsjoen P, Langsjoen P, Folkers K: Long-term efficacy and safety of coenzyme Q10 therapy for idiopathic dilated cardiomyopathy. *Am J Cardiol* 1990;65:521–523.

251. Engelsen J, Nielsen JD, Hansen KF: [Effect of coenzyme Q10 and ginkgo biloba on warfarin dosage in patients on long-term warfarin treatment: a randomized, double-blind, placebo-controlled cross-over trial.] [Article in Danish]. *Ugeskr Laeger* 2003;165:1868–1871.

252. Lamperti C, Naini AB, Lucchini V, et al.: Muscle coenzyme Q_{10} level in statin-related myopathy. *Arch Neurol* 2005;62:1709–1712.

253. Bleske BE, Willis RA, Anthony M, et al.: The effect of pravastatin and atorvastatin on coenzyme Q10. *Am Heart J* 2001;142:E2.

254. Mabuchi H, Higashikata T, Kawashiri M, et al.: Reduction of serum ubiquinol-10 and ubiquinone-10 levels by atorvastatin in hypercholesterolemic patients. *J Atheroscler Thromb* 2005;12:111–119.

255. Rundek T, Naini A, Sacco R, et al.: Atorvastatin decreases the coenzyme Q10 level in the blood of patients at risk for cardiovascular disease and stroke. *Arch Neurol* 2004;61:889–892.

256. Miyake Y, Shouzu A, Nishikawa M, et al.: Effect of treatment with 3-hydroxy-3-methylglutaryl coenzyme A reductase inhibitors on serum coenzyme Q10 in diabetic patients. *Arzneimittelforschung* 1999;49:324–329.

257. Iarussi D, Auricchio U, Agretto A, et al.: Protective effect of coenzyme Q10 on anthracycline cardiotoxicity: control study in children with acute lymphoblastic leukemia and non-Hodgkin's lymphoma. *Molec Aspects Med* 1994;15 (Suppl.):207–212.

258. Langsjoen P, Langsjoen P, Willis R, Folkers K: Treatment of essential hypertension with coenzyme Q10. *Molec Aspects Med* 1994;15 (Suppl.):165–172.

259. Singh RB, Niaz MA, Rastogi SS, Shukla PK, Thakur AS: Effect of hydrosoluble coenzyme Q10 on blood pressures and insulin resistance in hypertensive patients with coronary artery disease. *J Hum Hypertens* 1999;13:203–208.

260. Morisco C, Terimarco B, Condorelli M: Effect of coenzyme Q10 therapy in patients with congestive heart failure: a long-term multi-center randomized study. *Clin Invest* 1993;71:S134–S136.

261. Khatta M, Alexander BS, Krichten CM, Fisher ML, Freudenberger R, Robinson SW, Gottlieb SS: The effect of coenzyme Q10 in patients with congestive heart failure. *Ann Intern Med* 2000;132:636–640.

262. Mortensen SA: Overview on coenzyme Q10 as adjunctive therapy in chronic heart failure: rationale, design and end-points of "Q-symbio": a multinational trial. *Biofactors* 2003;18:79–89.

263. Henriksen JE, Andersen CB, Hother-Nielsen O, Vaag A, Aage Mortensen S, Beck-Nielsen H: Impact of ubiquinone (coenzyme Q10) treatment on glycaemic control, insulin requirement and well-being in patients with type 1 diabetes mellitus. *Diabetic Med* 1999;16:312–318.

264. Eriksson JG, Forsen TJ, Mortensen SA, Rohde M: The effect of coenzyme Q10 administration on metabolic control in patients with type 2 diabetes mellitus. *Biofactors* 1999;9:315–318.

265. Hodgson JM, Watts GF, Playford DA, et al.: Coenzyme Q10 improves blood pressure and glycaemic control: a controlled trial in subjects with type 2 diabetes. *Eur J Clin Nutr* 2002;56:1137–1142.

266. Nichols TW: Alpha-lipoic acid: biological effects and clinical implications. *Altern Med Rev* 1997;2:177–183.

267. Evans JL, Goldfine ID: Alpha-lipoic acid: a multi-functional antioxidant that improves insulin sensitivity in patients with type 2 diabetes. *Diabetes Technol Ther* 2000;2:401–413.

268. Packer L: Antioxidant properties of lipoic acid and its therapeutic effects in prevention of diabetes complications and cataracts. *Ann NY Acad Sci* 1994;738:257–264.

269. Giugliano D, Ceriello A, Paolisso G: Oxidative stress and diabetic vascular complications. *Diabetes Care* 1996;19:257–267.

270. Ziegler D: Thioctic acid for patients with symptomatic diabetic polyneuropathy: a critical review. *Treat Endocrinol* 2004;3:173–189.

271. Rudich A, Tirosh A, Potashnik R, Khamaisi M, Bashan N: Lipoic acid protects against oxidative stress induced impairment in insulin stimulation of protein kinase B and glucose transport in 3T3-L1 adipocytes. *Diabetologia* 1999;42:949–957.

272. Ziegler D, Hanefeld M, Ruhnau K-J, Meibner HP, Lobisch M, Schutte K, Gries FA, The ALADIN Study Group: Treatment of symptomatic diabetic peripheral neuropathy with the anti-oxidant "-lipoic acid: a 3-week multicentre randomized controlled trial (ALADIN Study I). *Diabetologia* 1995;38:1425–1433.

273. Reljanovic M, Reichel G, Rett K, Lobisch M, Schuette K, Moller W, Tritschler HJ, Mehnert H, ALADIN II Study Group: Treatment of diabetic polyneuropathy with the antioxidant thioctic acid (alpha-lipoic acid): a two year multicenter randomized double-blind placebo controlled trial (ALADIN II): Alpha Lipoid Acid in Diabetic Neuropathy. *Free Radic Biol Med* 1999;31:171–179.

274. Ziegler D, Hanefeld M, Ruhnau K-J, Hasche H, Lobisch M, Schutte K, Kerum G, Malessa R, ALADIN III Study Group: Treatment of symptomatic diabetic polyneuropathy with the antioxidant α-lipoic acid: a 7-month multicenter randomized controlled trial (ALADIN III Study). *Diabetes Care* 1999;22:1296–1301.

275. Ziegler D, Ametov A, Barinov A, et al.: Oral treatment with α-lipoic acid improves symptomatic diabetic neuropathy: the SYDNEY 2 trial. *Diabetes Care* 2006;29:2365–2370.

276. Ziegler D, Reljanovic M, Mehnert H, Gries FA: Alpha-lipoic acid in the treatment of diabetic polyneuropathy in Germany: current evidence from clinical trials. *Exp Clin Endocrinol Diabetes* 1999;107:421–430.

277. The SYDNEY Trial Study Group: The sensory symptoms of diabetic poly-neuropathy are improved with lipoic acid. *Diabetes Care* 2003;26:770–776.

278. Ziegler D, Nowak H, Kemplert P, et al.: Treatment of symptomatic diabetic polyneuropathy with the antioxidant α-lipoic acid: a meta-analysis. *Diabet Med* 2004;21:114–121.

279. Food and Nutrition Board, Institute of Medicine: *Dietary Reference Intakes for Vitamin C, Vitamin E, Selenium, and Carotenoids.* Washington, DC, National Academy Press, 2000. Available at http://www.nap.edu/books/0309069351/html.

280. Fryer MJ: Vitamin E as a protective antioxidant in progressive renal failure. *Nephrology* 2000;5:1–7.

281. Lonn E, Bosch J, Yusuf S, et al.: Effects of long-term vitamin E supplementation on cardiovascular events and cancer: a randomized controlled trial. *JAMA* 2005;293:1338–1347.

282. Miller ER III, Pastor-Barriuso R, Dalal D, et al.: Meta-analysis: high-dosage vitamin E supplementation may increase all-cause mortality. *Ann Intern Med* 2005;142:37–46.

283. Helson L: The effect of intravenous vitamin E and menadiol sodium diphosphate on vitamin K dependent clotting factors. *Throm Res* 1984; 35:11–18.

284. Brown BG, Zhao XQ, Chait A: Simvastatin and niacin, antioxidant vitamins, or the combination for the prevention of coronary disease. *N Engl J Med* 2001;345:1583–1593.

285. Paolisso G, D'Amore A, Galzzerano D, et al.: Daily vitamin E supplements improve metabolic control but not insulin secretion in elderly type 2 diabetes patients. *Diabetes Care* 1993;11:1433–1437.

286. Alpha-Tocopherol, Beta Carotene Cancer Prevention Study Group: The effect of vitamin E and beta carotene on the incidence of lung cancer and other cancers in male smokers. *N Engl J Med* 1994;330:1029–1035.

287. Stephens NG, Parsons A, Schofield PM, et al.: Randomised controlled trial of vitamin E in patients with coronary disease: Cambridge Heart Antioxidant Study: CHAOS. *Lancet* 1996;347:781–786.

288. Gruppo Italiano per lo Studio della Sopravvivenza nell'Infarto miocardico (GISSI Prevenzione Investigators): Dietary supplementation with n-3 polyunsaturated fatty acids and vitamin E after myocardial infarction: results of the GISSI-Prevenzione trial. *Lancet* 1999;354:447–455.

289. Yusuf S, Dagenais G, Pogue J, et al.: Vitamin E supplementation and cardiovascular events in high-risk patients: the Heart Outcomes Prevention Evaluation study. *N Engl J Med* 2000;342:154–160.

290. Heart Protection Study Collaborative Group: MRC/BHF Heart Protection Study of antioxidant vitamin supplementation in 20,536 high-risk individuals: a randomized placebo-controlled trial. *Lancet* 2002;360: 23–33.

291. Ford ES, Ajani UA, Mokdad AH: Brief communication: the prevalence of high intake of vitamin E from the use of supplements among U.S. adults. *Ann Intern Med* 2005;143:116–120.

292. Tribble DL: AHA science advisory: antioxidant consumption and risk of coronary heart disease: emphasis on vitamin C, vitamin E, and beta-carotene: a statement for healthcare professionals from the American Heart Association. *Circulation* 1999;99:591–595.

293. Jiang Q, Christen S, Shigenaga MK, Ames BN: γ-Tocopherol, the major form of vitamin E in the US diet, deserves more attention. *Am J Clin Nutr* 2001;74:714–722.

294. Robinson I, de Serna DG, Gutierrez A, Schade DS: Vitamin E in humans: an explanation of clinical trial failure. *Endocr Pract* 2006;12:576–582.

295. Jamal GA: The use of gamma linolenic acid in the prevention and treatment of diabetic neuropathy. *Diabet Med* 1994;11:145–149.

296. Jamal GA, Carmichael H: The effect of gamma-linolenic acid on human diabetic peripheral neuropathy: a double-blind placebo-controlled trial. *Diabet Med* 1990;7:319–323.

297. Keen H, Payan J, Allawi J, et al.: Treatment of diabetic neuropathy with gamma-linolenic acid: the Gamma-Linolenic Acid Multicenter Trial Group. *Diabetes Care*. 1993;16:8–15.

298. Horrobin DF: Essential fatty acids in the management of impaired nerve function in diabetes. *Diabetes* 1997;46:S90–S93.

299. Purewal TS, Evans PMS, Havard F, O'Hare JP: Lack of effect of evening primrose oil on autonomic function tests after 12 months of treatment (Abstract). *Diabetologia* 1997;40 (Suppl. 1):A556.

300. Kleijnen J, Knipschild P: Ginkgo biloba. *Lancet* 1992;340:1136–1139.

301. Ritch R: Complementary therapy for the treatment of glaucoma: a perspective. *Ophthalmol Clin North Am* 2005;18:597–609.

302. Bent S, Goldberg H, Padula A, Avins AL: Spontaneous bleeding associated with ginkgo biloba: a case report and systematic review of the literature. *J Gen Intern Med* 2005;20:657–661.

303. Galluzzi S, Zanetti O, Binetti G, Trabucchi M, Frisoni GB: Coma in a patient with Alzheimer's disease taking low dose trazodone and gingko biloba. *J Neurol Neurosurg Psychiatry* 2000;68:679–680.

304. Markowitz JS, Donovan JL, DeVane L, et al.: Multiple dose administration of ginkgo biloba did not affect cytochrome P-450 2D6 or 3A4 activity in normal volunteers. *J Clin Psychopharmacol* 2003;23:576–581.

305. Kudolo GB: The effect of 3-month ingestion of ginkgo biloba extract on pancreatic beta-cell function in response to glucose loading in normal glucose tolerant individuals. *J Clin Pharmacol* 2000;40:647–654.

306. Kudolo GB: The effect of 3-month ingestion of gingko biloba extract (EGb 761) on pancreatic beta-cell function in response to glucose loading in individuals with non-insulin-dependent diabetes mellitus. *J Clin Pharmacol* 2001;41:600–611.

307. Kudolo GB, Wang W, Elrod R, et al.: Short-term ingestion of ginkgo biloba extract does not alter whole body insulin sensitivity in non-diabetic, pre-diabetic or type 2 diabetic subjects: a randomized double-blind placebo-controlled crossover study. *Clin Nutr* 2006;25:123–134.

308. Peters H, Kieser M, Holscher U: Demonstration of the efficacy of ginkgo biloba special extract EGb 761 on intermittent claudication: a placebo-controlled double-blind multicenter trial. *Vasa* 1998;27:106–110.

309. Pittler MH, Ernst E: Ginkgo biloba extract for the treatment of intermittent claudication: a meta analysis of randomized trials. *Am J Med.* 2000;108:276–281.

310. Horsch S, Walther C: Ginkgo biloba special extract EGb761 in the treatment of peripheral arterial occlusive disease (PAOD): a review based on randomized controlled studies. *Int J Clin Pharmacol Ther* 2004;42:63–72.

311. Huang SY, Jeng C, Kao SC, et al.: Improved haemorrheological properties by ginkgo biloba extract (EGb 761) in type 2 diabetes mellitus complicated with retinopathy. *Clin Nutr* 2004;23:615–621.

312. Kris-Etherton PM, Harris WS, Appel LJ, Nutrition Committee: Fish consumption, fish oil, omega-3 fatty acids, and cardiovascular disease. *Circulation* 2002;106:2747–2757.

313. Oh R: Practical applications of fish oil (Ω-3 fatty acids) in primary care. *J Am Board Fam Pract* 2005;18:28–36.

314. Ruxton CHS, Reed SC, Simpson MJA, Millington KJ: The health benefits of omega-3 polyunsaturated fatty acids: a review of the evidence. *J Hum Nutr Dietet* 2004;17:449–459.

315. Nettleton JA, Katz R: N-3 long-chain polyunsaturated fatty acids in type 2 diabetes: a review. *J Am Diet Assoc* 2005;105:428–440.

316. Marchioli R, Barzi F, Bomba E, et al.: Early protection against sudden death by n-3 polyunsaturated fatty acids after myocardial infarction: time course analysis of the results of the Gruppo Italiano per lo Studio della Sopravvivenza nell'Infarto Miocardico (GISSI)-Prevenzione. *Circulation* 2002;105:1897–1903.

317. Farmer A, Montori V, Dinneen S, Clar C: Fish oil in people with type 2 diabetes mellitus. *Cochrane Database of Systematic Reviews* 2001, Issue 3. Art. No.: CD003205. doi:10.1002/14651858.CD003205.

318. Friedberg CE, Jannsen MJEM, Heine RJ, Grobbee DE: Fish oil and glycemic control in diabetes. *Diabetes Care* 1998;21:494–500.

319. Montori VM, Farmer A, Wollan PC, Dinneen SF: Fish oil supplementation in type 2 diabetes, a quantitative systemic review. *Diabetes Care* 2000;23:1407–1415.

320. Studer M, Matthias B, Leimenstoll B, et al.: Effect of different antilipidemic agents and diets on mortality. *Arch Intern Med* 2005;165:725–730.

321. American Diabetes Association: Nutrition recommendations and interventions for diabetes—2006 (Position Statement). *Diabetes Care* 2006;29:2140–2157

322. MacLean CH, Mojica WA, Morton SC, et al.: Effects of omega-3 fatty acids on lipids and glycemic control in type II diabetes and the metabolic syndrome and on inflammatory bowel disease, rheumatoid arthritis, renal disease, systemic lupus erythematosus, and osteoporosis. Summary, Evidence Report/Technology Assessment No. 89. (Prepared by the Southern California/RAND Evidence-based Practice Center, Los Angeles, CA.) AHRQ Publication No. 04-E012-1. Rockville, Md., Agency for Healthcare Research and Quality, March 2004.

323. Omacor package insert. Available at http://www.fda.gov/cder/foi/label/2004/21654lbl.pdf. Accessed July 8, 2006.

324. Pepping J: Policosanol. *Am J Health-Syst Pharm* 2003;60:1112–1114.

325. Anonymous: Policosanol. *Altern Med Rev* 2004;9:312–317.

326. Gouni-Berthold I, Berthold HK: Policosanol: clinical pharmacology and therapeutic significance of a new lipid-lowering agent. *Am Heart J* 2002;143:356–365.

327. Torres O, Agramonte AJ, Illnait J, et al.: Treatment of hypercholesterolemia in NIDDM with policosanol. *Diabetes Care* 1995;18:393–397.

328. Crespo N, Illnait J, Mas R, et al.: Comparative study of the efficacy and tolerability of policosanol and lovastatin in patients with hypercholesterolemia and noninsulin dependent diabetes mellitus. *Int J Clin Pharmacol Res* 1999;19:117–127.

329. Chen JT, Wesley R, Shamburek RD, et al.: Meta-analysis of natural therapies for hyperlipidemia: plant sterols and stanols versus policosanol. *Pharmacotherapy* 2005;25:171–183.

330. Berthold HK, Unverdorben S, Degenhardt R, Bulitta M, Gouni-Berthold I: Effect of policosanol on lipid levels among patients with hypercholesterolemia or combined hyperlipidemia, a randomized controlled trial. *JAMA* 2006;295:2262–2269.

331. Canetti M, Moreira M, Mas R, et al.: A two-year study on the efficacy and tolerability of policosanol in patients with type II hyperlipoproteinaemia. *Int J Clin Pharmacol Res* 1995;15:159–165.

332. Castano G, Mas R, Fernandez L, et al.: A long-term study of policosanol in the treatment of intermittent claudication. *Angiology* 2001;52:1115–1125.

333. Lin Y, Rudrum M, Van Der Wielen RP, et al.: Wheat germ policosanol failed to lower plasma cholesterol in subjects with normal to mildly elevated cholesterol concentrations. *Metabolism* 2004;53:1309–1314.

334. Castano G, Mas R, Fernandez L, et al.: Comparison of the efficacy and tolerability of policosanol with atorvastatin in elderly patients with type II hypercholesterolaemia. *Drugs Aging* 2003;20:153–163.

335. Tattelman E: Health effects of garlic. *Am Fam Physician* 2005;72:103–106.

336. Ackermann RT, Mulrow CD, et al.: Garlic shows promise for improving some cardiovascular risk factors. *Arch Intern Med* 2001;161:813–814.

337. Pareddy SR, Rosenberg JM: Does garlic have useful medicinal purposes? *Hosp Pharm Rep* 1993;8:27.

338. Stevinson C, Pittler MH, Ernst E: Garlic for treating hypercholesterolemia, a meta-analysis of randomized clinical trials. *Ann Intern Med* 2000;133:420–429.

339. Ashraf R, Aamir K, Shaikh AR, Ahmed T: Effects of garlic on dyslipidemia in patients with type 2 diabetes mellitus. *J Ayub Med Coll Abbottabad* 2005;17:60–64.

340. Silagy CA, Neil HA: A meta-analysis of the effect of garlic on blood pressure. *J Hypertens* 1994;12:463–468.

341. Ahmad MS, Ahmed M: Antiglycation properties of aged garlic extract: possible role in prevention of diabetic complications. *J Nutr* 2006;136 (3 Suppl.):796S–799S.

342. Shields KM, Moranville MP: Guggul for hypercholesterolemia. *Am J Health-Syst Pharm* 2005;62:1012–1014.

343. Singh RB, Niaz MA, Ghosh S: Hypolipidemic and antioxidant effects of *Commiphora mukul* as an adjunct to dietary therapy in patients with hypercholesterolemia. *Cardiovasc Drugs Ther* 1994;8:659–664.

344. Szapary PO, Wolfe ML, Bloedon LT, et al.: Guggulipid for the treatment of hypercholesterolemia, a randomized controlled trial. *JAMA* 2003;290:765–772.

345. Sahni S, Hepfinger CA, Sauer KA: Guggulipid use in hyperlipidemia: case report and review of the literature. *Am J Health-Syst Pharm* 2005;62:1690–1692.

346. Anonymous: *Monascus purpureus* (red yeast rice). *Altern Med Rev* 2004; 9:208–210.

347. Heber D, Yip I, Ashley JM, et al.: Cholesterol-lowering effects of a proprietary Chinese red-yeast-rice dietary supplement. *Am J Clin Nutr* 1999;69:231–236.

348. Bladt S, Wagner H: Inhibition of MAO by fractions and constituents of hypericum extract. *J Geriatr Psychiatry Neurol* 1994;7:S57–S59.

349. Muller WE: Current St John's wort research from mode of action to clinical efficacy. *Pharmacol Res* 2003;47:101–109.

350. Lawvere S, Mahoney MC: St. John's wort. *Am Fam Physician* 2005; 72:2249–2254.

351. Gulick RM, McAuliffe V, Holden-Wiltse J, et al.: Phase I studies of hypericin, the active compound in St John's wort, as an antiretroviral agent in HIV-infected adults. *Ann Intern Med* 1999;130:510–514.

352. Beckman SE, Sommi RW, Switzer J: Consumer use of St John's wort: a survey on effectiveness, safety, and tolerability. *Pharmacotherapy* 2000;20:568–574.

353. Ferko N, Levine MA: Evaluation of the association between St John's wort and elevated thyroid-stimulating hormone. *Pharmacotherapy* 2001;21:1574–1578.

354. Hauben M: The association of St John's wort with elevated thyroid-stimulating hormone. *Pharmacotherapy* 2002;22:673–675.

355. Schulz V: Safety of St. John's wort extract compared to synthetic antidepressants. *Phytomedicine* 2006;13:199–204.

356. Lantz MS, Buchalter DO, Giambanco V: St John's wort and antidepressant drug interactions in the elderly. *J Geriatr Psychiatry Neurol* 1999;12:7–10.

357. Zhou S, Chan E, Pan S-Q, Huang M, Lee EJD: Pharmacokinetic interactions of drugs with St. John's wort. *J Psychopharmacol* 2004;18:262–276.

358. Linde K, Mulrow CD: St John's wort for depression. *Cochrane Reviews* [computer software]. Oxford, U.K., The Cochrane Library, Update software, 2000.

359. Woelk H: Comparison of St John's wort and imipramine for treating depression: randomized controlled trial. *BMJ* 2000;321:536–539.

360. Shrader E: Equivalence of St John's wort (ZE117) and fluoxetine: a randomized, controlled study in mild-moderate depression. *Int Clin Psychopharmacol* 2000;15:61–68.

361. Brenner R, Azbel V, Madhusoodanan S, Pawlowska M: Comparison of an extract of hypericum (LI 160) and sertraline in the treatment of depression: a double-blind, randomized pilot study. *Clin Ther* 2000;22:411–419.

362. Shelton RC, Keller MB, Gelenberg A, et al.: Effectiveness of St John's wort in major depression; a randomized control trial. *JAMA* 2001;285:1978–1986.

363. Hypericum Depression Trial Study Group: Effect of *Hypericum perforatum* (St John's wort) in major depressive disorder: a randomized controlled trial. *JAMA* 2002;287:1807–1814.

364. Szegedi A, Kohnen R, Dienel A, Kieser M: Acute treatment of moderate to severe depression with hypericum extract WS5570 (St John's wort): randomised controlled double blind non-inferiority trial versus paroxetine. *BMJ* doi:10.1136/bmj.38356.655266.82 (published online 11 February 2005).

365. Fava M, Alpert J, Nierenberg AA, et al.: A double-blind, randomized trial of St. John's wort, fluoxetine, and placebo in major depressive disorder. *J Clin Psychopharmacol* 2005;25:441–447.

366. Yeh GY, Eisenberg DM, Kaptchuk TJ, Phillips RS: Systematic review of herbs and dietary supplements for glycemic control in diabetes. *Diabetes Care.* 2003;26:1277–1294.

367. U.S. Preventive Services Task Force: *Guide to Clinical Preventive Services: An Assessment of the Effectiveness of 169 Interventions.* Baltimore, MD, Williams & Wilkins, 1989.

368. American Diabetes Association: Standards of medical care for patients with diabetes (Position Statement). *Diabetes Care.* 2007;30 (Suppl. 1):S4–S41.

369. Mingrone G: Carnitine in type 2 diabetes. *Ann NY Acad Sci* 2004;1033:99–107.

370. Mingrone G, Greco AV, Capristo E, et al.: L-carnitine improves glucose disposal in type 2 diabetic patients. *J Am Coll Nutr* 1999;18:77–82.

371. Rahbar AR, Shakerhosseini R, Saadat N, et al.: Effect of L-carnitine on plasma glycemic and lipidemic profile in patients with type II diabetes mellitus. *Eur J Clin Nutr* 2005;59:592–596.

372. De Grandis D, Minardi C: Acetyl-L-carnitine (levacecarnine) in the treatment of diabetic neuropathy: a long-term, randomised, double-blind, placebo-controlled study. *Drugs R D* 2002;3:223–231.

373. Sima AA, Calvani M, Mehra M, Amato A, Acetyl-L-Carnitine Study Group: Acetyl-L-Carnitine improves pain, nerve regeneration and vibratory perception in patients with chronic diabetic neuropathy: an analysis of two randomized placebo-controlled trials. *Diabetes Care* 2005;28:89–94.

374. Grassi D, Lippi C, Necozione S, Desideri F, Ferri C: Short-term administration of dark chocolate is followed by a significant increase in insulin sensitivity and a decrease in blood pressure in healthy persons. *Am J Clin Nutr* 2005;81:611–614.

375. Grassi D, Necozione S, Lippi C, et al.: Cocoa reduces blood pressure and insulin resistance and improves endothelium-dependent vasodilation in hypertensives. *Hypertension* 2005;46:398–405.

376. Keen CL, Holt RR, Oteiza PI, Fraga CG, Schmitz HH: Cocoa antioxidants and cardiovascular health. *Am J Clin Nutr* 2005;81(1 Suppl.):298S–303S.

377. Hoodia. Available at http://en.wikipedia.org/wiki/Hoodia. Accessed January 22, 2007.

378. American Diabetes Association. Unproven therapies (Position Statement). *Diabetes Care.* 2003;26:S142.

Bibliography and Useful Websites for Clinicians

Jellin JM, Gregory PJ, Batz F, Hitchens K, et al.: *Pharmacist's Letter/Prescribers Letter NaturalMedicines Comprehensive Database.* 9th ed. Stockton, Calif., Therapeutic Research Faculty, 2007.

DerMarderosian A, Beutler JA, Eds.: *The Review of Natural Products.* St. Louis, Mo., Wolters Kluwer Health, 2006.

Fetrow CW, Avila JR, Eds.: *Professional's Handbook of Complementary and Alternative Medicines.* 3rd ed. Springhouse, Penn., Lippincott Williams & Wilkins, 2004.

Sarubin Fragakis A: *The Health Professional's Guide to Popular Dietary Supplements.* 2nd ed. Chicago, American Dietetic Association, 2003.

Haggans CJ, Regan KS, Brown LM, et al.: Computer access to research on dietary supplements: a database of federally funded dietary supplement research. *J Nutr* 2005;135:1796–1799.

National Institutes of Health National Center for Complementary and Alternative Medicine (NCCAM). Available at http://www.nccam.nih.gov.

U.S. Pharmacopeia (USP). Available at http://www.usp.org.

Link to Dietary Supplements at the Food and Nutrition Information Center. U.S. Department of Agriculture Agricultural Research Service, National Agricultural Library. Available at http://fnic.nal.usda.gov/nal_display/index.php?info_center = 4&tax_level = 1&tax_subject = 274.

International Bibliographic Information on Dietary Supplements (IBIDS) Database. National Institutes of Health Office of Dietary Supplements. Available at http://ods.od.nih.gov/Health_Information/IBIDS.aspx.

"Tips for the Savvy Supplement User: Making Informed Decisions and Evaluating Information." Available at http://www.cfsan.fda.gov/-dms/ds-savvy.html.

"Tips for Older Dietary Supplement Users." Available at http://www.cfsan.fda.gov/-dms/ds-savv2.html.

Index

Guggul (*Commiphora mukul*), 136
Gymnema (*Gymnema sylvestre R. Br.*), 18, 75
   adverse effects of, 19

Hamburg Pain Adjective List, 113
Harris Poll, 11
The Health Professional's Guide to Popular Dietary Supplements, 13
hepatotoxic drugs
   and effect of milk thistle, 74
Hispanics, with diabetes, 8, 9
holy basil (*Ocimum sanctum*), 41, 79, 80
   chemical constituents and action mechanism of, 41
   effects of consumption, 42
Hoodia gordonii Masson, 158
Hoodia, appetite-suppressant effects, 159
hyperforin, 5
hypericin, 5
hyperlipidemia
   role of Guar gum, 56, 57
hypermagnesemia, 98
hypomagnesemia, 97, 100

Indian kino tree, 43
   product of bark, 45
insulin activity, 88
insulin receptor or β-cell sensitivity
   impact of chromium on, 89
irreversible hypoglycemia, 4
Islet cell antibodies (ICAs), 95
ispaghula husk. *See* Blonde psyllium
Ivy gourd (*Coccinia indica*), 38, 79
   side effects of, 39
   chemical constituents and action mechanism of, 38, 39
   efficacy in treatment of diabetes, 40

jambolan (*Eugenia jambolana or Syzygium cumini*), 45, 81
   an ingredient in multi-ingredient dietary supplements, 47
   chemical constituents and action mechanism of, 45, 46

konjac flour, 51
konjac mannan. *See* Glucomannan
Kuna Indians, 158

L-carnitine, 157, 158
leguminosae family, Fenugreek, 21
lipid-lowering agents, 55. *See also* Guar gum
lipoperoxidation
   impact on diabetic pateints, 72
L-β-hydroxy-γ-N-trimethylamino-butyric acid, 157

madhu meha, 18
magnesium, 109
   adverse effects of, 97, 98
   as antacid, 97
   mechanism of action, 97
magnesium deficiency, 97
   and type 2 diabetes, 100
magnesium depleting medications, 100
magnesium intake
   and risk of type 2 diabetes, 98, 99
magnesium toxicity, 100
Medical Expenditure Panel Survey, 1996, 8
Metamucil, 50. *See also* blonde psyllium
milk thistle (*Silybum marianum*), 71, 86
   chemical constituents and action mechanism of, 71, 72
   side effects of, 72, 73
   used for nonalcoholic steatohepatitis, 74

spironolactone, 98

St. John's wort (*Hypericum perforatum* L.),
    141, 155
    adverse effects, 142–143
    and marker constituents, 5
    uses, 144–145

Stephania tetranda, 5

Stevia (*Stevia rebaudiana Bertoni*), 57, 83
    as noncaloric sweetener, 59, 60
    chemical constituents and action
        mechanism of, 57, 58
    primary adverse effects of, 58

Sweet ex Decne, 158

SYDNEY trials, 114

synthetic vitamin E, 116

Tea (*Camellia sinensis*), 64, 84
    chemical constituents and action
        mechanism of, 65
    main adverse effects of, 65–66
    popular beverage, 67
    types of, 64

teratogenicity, 93

Theaceae family, 64

tinctures, 4

tulsi. See holy basil

U.S. Pharmacopeia (USP), 11, 163

U.S. Preventive Services Task Force
    criteria, 157

Ubiquinone. *See* Coenzyme Q10

USP-verified mark, 11

vanadis. *See* Vanadium

Vanadium, 107, 108
    average intake of, 91
    mechanism of action, 92
    side effects of, 92

vanadium supplements, usage by diabetic
    patients, 93

Vietnamese population, with diabetes, 8

Vijayasar (*Pterocarpus marsupium Roxb.*),
    43, 45, 80. *See also* Indian kino
    tree
    chemical constituents and action
        mechanism of, 41

Vitamin B. *See* Nicotinamide

Vitamin E, 147
    adverse effects and drug interactions,
        116–117
    chemical constituents and mechanism
        of action, 116
    clinical studies, 117–118
    consumption rates, 118
    dietary intake recommendations, 119
    uses of, 118

Warfarin (Coumadin), 21

water-based CAM supplements,
    4

weight-loss supplement, 157. *See also*
    CAM supplements

Other Titles Available from the American Diabetes Association

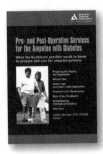

Pre- and Post-Operative Services for the Diabetic Amputee
by Sander A. Nassan, CPO
Great effort is put into avoiding the diabetes complications that lead to amputation, but despite best efforts, it still happens. In this volume, Nassan et al. give you the necessary tools to help patients face the trauma of amputation, including identifying the needs of the amputee, prescribing physical therapy, and identifying a patient's learning style.
Order no. 5429-01; Price $49.95

Therapy for Diabetes Mellitus and Related Disorders, 4th Edition
edited by Harold E. Lebovitz
Deliver proven treatments to your patients with this new edition of an essential book. Leading diabetes experts around the world provide a concise overview of the new advances in and an update on diabetes therapy, including glycemic control, type 2 diabetes prevention, diabetes in pregnancy, insulin pump therapy, and oral and cardiovascular disease.
Order no. 5402-04; Price $59.95

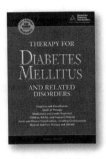

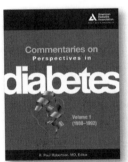

Commentaries on Perspectives in Diabetes
edited by R. Paul Robertson, MD
In this three-volume set, the original authors of many of the popular Perspectives in Diabetes articles published in the journal *Diabetes* revisit their original work and discuss what has changed over the past 18 years. Discover how the authors have given new life to their ideas, ensuring further and better development of new and effective therapies for diabetes.
Volume 1: Order no. 5430-01; Price $ 49.95
Volume 2: Order no. 5431-01; Price $ 49.95
Volume 3: Order no. 5432-01; Price $ 49.95
Complete Set: Order no. 6064-18; Price $104.95

Practical Insulin, 2nd Edition
by American Diabetes Association
This indispensable resource will give you the knowledge and data you need for initiating and maintaining insulin therapy in patients with type 1 or type 2 diabetes. Find fast, current, reliable information on insulin regimens, starting doses, correcting doses, insulin analogs, inhaled insulin, and matching insulin regimens to patients. With this easy reference guide, you can make improved glycemic control an attainable reality for your patients.

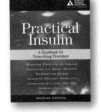

Order no. 5420-02; Price $7.95

About the American Diabetes Association

The American Diabetes Association is the nation's leading voluntary health organization supporting diabetes research, information, and advocacy. Its mission is to prevent and cure diabetes and to improve the lives of all people affected by diabetes. The American Diabetes Association is the leading publisher of comprehensive diabetes information. Its huge library of practical and authoritative books for people with diabetes covers every aspect of self-care—cooking and nutrition, fitness, weight control, medications, complications, emotional issues, and general self-care.

To order American Diabetes Association books: Call 1-800-232-6733 or log on to *http://store.diabetes.org*

To join the American Diabetes Association: Call 1-800-806-7801 or log on to *www. diabetes.org/membership*

For more information about diabetes or ADA programs and services: Call 1-800-342-2383. E-mail: AskADA@diabetes.org or log on to *www.diabetes.org*

To locate an ADA/NCQA Recognized Provider of quality diabetes care in your area: *www.ncqa.org/dprp*

To find an ADA Recognized Education Program in your area: Call 1-800-342-2383. *www.diabetes.org/for-health-professionals-and-scientists/recognition/edrecognition.jsp*

To join the fight to increase funding for diabetes research, end discrimination, and improve insurance coverage: Call 1-800-342-2383. *www.diabetes.org/advocacy-and-legalresources/advocacy.jsp*

To find out how you can get involved with the programs in your community: Call 1-800-342-2383. See below for program Web addresses.

- *American Diabetes Month:* educational activities aimed at those diagnosed with diabetes—month of November. *www.diabetes.org/communityprograms-and-localevents/ americandiabetesmonth.jsp*

- *American Diabetes Alert:* annual public awareness campaign to find the undiagnosed—held the fourth Tuesday in March. *www.diabetes.org/communityprograms-and-localevents/ americandiabetesalert.jsp*

- *American Diabetes Association Latino Initiative:* diabetes awareness program targeted to the Latino community. *www.diabetes.org/communityprograms-and-localevents/latinos.jsp*

- *African American Program:* diabetes awareness program targeted to the African American community. *www.diabetes.org/communityprograms-and-localevents/africanamericans.jsp*

- *Awakening the Spirit: Pathways to Diabetes Prevention & Control:* diabetes awareness program targeted to the Native American community. *www.diabetes.org/ communityprograms-and-localevents/nativeamericans.jsp*

To find out about an important research project regarding type 2 diabetes: *www.diabetes.org/diabetes-research/research-home.jsp*

To obtain information on making a planned gift or charitable bequest: Call 1-888-700-7029. *www.wpg.cc/stl/CDA/homepage/1,1006,509,00.html*

To make a donation or memorial contribution: Call 1-800-342-2383. *www.diabetes.org/support-the-cause/make-a-donation.jsp*

▲. American Diabetes Association®

Cure • Care • Commitment®